Second Edition

Drug Dosage Calculations

WITHDRAWN

A Guide for Clinical Practice

Geraldine Ann Medici, M.S., R.N., C.S.
Associate Professor of Nursing
Northeastern University
Boston, Massachusetts

10-91   Gift

APPLETON & LANGE
Norwalk, Connecticut/San Mateo, California

0-8385-1775-7

Copyright © 1988 by Appleton & Lange
A Publishing Division of Prentice Hall
Copyright © 1980 by Prentice-Hall, Inc.

88 89 90 91 92 / 10 9 8 7 6 5 4 3 2 1

Prentice-Hall of Australia, Pty. Ltd., Sydney
Prentice-Hall Canada, Inc.
Prentice-Hall Hispanoamericana, S.A., Mexico
Prentice-Hall of India Private Limited, New Delhi
Prentice-Hall International (UK) Limited, London
Prentice-Hall of Japan, Inc., Tokyo
Prentice-Hall of Southeast Asia (Pte.) Ltd., Singapore
Whitehall Books Ltd., Wellington, New Zealand
Editora Prentice-Hall do Brasil Ltda., Rio de Janeiro

Library of Congress Cataloging-in-Publication Data

Medici, Geraldine Ann.
  Drug dosage calculations.

  1. Pharmaceutical arithmetic. 2. Drugs—Dosage.
I. Title. [DNLM: 1. Drugs—administration & dosage.
QV 748 M489d]
RS57.M43   1988   615'.14   87-19455
ISBN 0-8385-1775-7

Production Editor: Karen W. Davis
Designer: M. Chandler Martylewski
Cover design by Steven Byrum

PRINTED IN THE UNITED STATES OF AMERICA

To the Second Edition

Life teaches us many things, one being that things are always changing and some things never change. With this in mind once again I start off my dedication with a grateful thank you to my family—Jackie, without you my revision goals would never have been reached—and end my dedication with an acknowledgment to my students, who continue to identify learning needs and serve as a test ground to prove my ideas work in meeting their learning needs.

To the First Edition

First and foremost, to my family without whom my abilities would never have been developed and nurtured; then to Elaine and Tom, who provided the stimulus; to my Dean and course group, who offered colleagueal support; to Philip, who gave me encouragement and understanding throughout this undertaking; to Terrie, who enabled me to meet my deadline; and finally, to my students, who proved my ideas worked and made the task worthwhile: A grateful thank you for assisting me in achieving my goal.

Contents

Preface

This book will develop the reader's competence in calculating drug dosages. The mathematical component of the administration of medication is presented in as complete a form as possible. Using class-tested material, and computer-analyzed test questions as a basis in its development, the presentation proceeds from the simple to the complex.

In Part I, you will find a self-assessment math test. It tests all the mathematical skills required for calculating drug dosages, and enables you to identify the specific areas that you need to review further. If review is indicated, you are advised to complete the appropriate sections of the basic/general mathematics review located in Chapter 3 before proceeding to Part II.

Part II covers the great variety of mathematical situations that you may encounter during the administration of medications. The emphasis is on metric measures, but in-depth practice with apothecary measures has also been included for those of you who practice in settings that still use both systems interchangeably. Because of the decreasing use of the apothecary system to measure drugs, practice related to this system is located in the last four chapters, Part III.

The organizational components of most chapters are as follows: (1) performance objectives; (2) a pretest; (3) text with example problems and activity,/practice sheets; (4) a posttest; and (5) an answer sheet. The format is programmed to structure learning, providing ample practice and immediate feedback to verify progress and stimulate further progression.

Specific performance objectives stated at the beginning of each chapter enable you to identify previously learned material. You may test this knowledge by taking the pretest. Each pretest question is keyed to the relevant performance objective(s) for ease in identification. This will assist you in deciding whether to focus on specific material in the current chapter, or to bypass the chapter and progress to new areas or chapters.

The text describes problem-solving techniques with the use of a few essential facts. The author has avoided long lists and tables. The content is arranged in a fashion that is easy to memorize, study, and review. Numerous example problems illustrate the use of facts, guides, and rules. The activity sheet, one for each section of text, contains questions/practice problems on material just presented and learned. Your answers should be checked against those listed at the end of the chapter, and errors corrected before proceeding to the next section. At the end of the chapter is a posttest to measure mastery of the stated objectives so that you can match any errors to the areas in which you need review. If you pass the posttest, you are ready to go on to the next chapter.

Because this book is a self-contained learning module, it allows you to progress at your own pace, and master the contents without assistance. It can be used, however, within a planned curriculum in various ways: in conjunction with formal/structured classes or without formal classes but requiring that the instructor set up a completion time schedule, tutor only those students who need assistance, and give an in-class final exam to verify achievement.

Completeness and flexibility make this book useful to a varied population. It is a basic in-depth preparatory tool for anyone who will be administering medicines. It is a review and reference book for upper level students, those who are studying for the State Board examination, and individuals already in or reentering the clinical setting. Finally, it can be used as a hospital in-service tool/reference to maintain or upgrade personal competency.

Geraldine Ann Medici

**Preparing to Master Drug
Dosage Calculations**

1

*Introductory Directions to
the Reader*

This book contains all the necessary information you need to calculate drug dosages. You can progress at your own rate of learning until you master the contents. The structure of this book will help you to master this material without assistance.

You are advised in most instances to follow the chapter sequence, as the material covered progresses in difficulty from simple to complex, and mastery of subsequent chapters is dependent upon knowledge and skills acquired in earlier chapters.

The chapters are grouped into three parts: Part I contains a self-assessment mathematics test specifically designed to test your competence in the mathematical skills that are necessary for calculating drug dosages. Compute all the problems before you correct this test. If you encounter difficulty with the self-assessment mathematics test, you are advised to complete the mathematics review in Chapter 3 before continuing to Part II. Part II covers most of the mathematical situations encountered in drug dosage calculations.

FORMAT

The format of each of the chapters in Parts II and III includes essentially (1) learning objectives, (2) a pretest, (3) text with example problems and activity/practice sheets, (4) a posttest, and (5) an answer sheet.

1. The *learning objectives* for each chapter are of two types: terminal performance objectives (TPO), and intermediate performance objectives (IPO). Terminal performance objectives state what behavioral skills you will learn to perform in the specific chapter or, in other words, what you should be capable of doing when you have completed the

chapter. The intermediate performance objectives are more specific and state the activities you must be able to perform in order to meet the terminal performance objectives. Intermediate performance objectives are the individual steps involved in reaching the terminal or ultimate objectives.

2. The *pretest* does not have to be taken by the novice. The pretest is specifically designed to verify mastery of the objectives of the chapter. If after reading the objectives, you feel that you know the material from previous experience, then take the pretest. If you calculate all the problems correctly, you may bypass that chapter, and continue to the next one and start the same process again. This allows the person with previous experience to accelerate. If you do not pass the pretest, start the chapter by reading, understanding, and memorizing the text.

3. The *activity sheet* is composed of questions, fill-ins, and problem-solving items. It provides structured practice that facilitates achievement of performance objectives of the chapter. After completing the activity sheet compare your answers with those listed at the end of the chapter. Remember, the aim is mastery of learning—100% accuracy. If any of your answers are incorrect, review the text and compute the incorrect items again before you go on.

4. When you have finished all the text and activity sheets in the chapter, you are ready for the *posttest*, which measures your achievement of the objectives established for the chapter. You will note TPO/IPO 1, 2, 3, . . . to the left of the test items on both the pretest and the posttest: this signifies the relationship between the test item and the performance objective(s) of the chapter. These letters and numbers will tell you which objectives you have and have not met. If you have met them all, you are ready to progress to the next chapter. If any of your computations have been inaccurate, review the text, return to the appropriate activity sheets for more practice, and then correct the posttest. When you have done this take the pretest as a second posttest. (The pretest and posttest are identical in structure.) When you have attained complete accuracy, you have assured mastery of that chapter, and you are ready to proceed to the next one.

5. All of the *answers* for each chapter appear at the end of the respective chapter.

You are encouraged to study alone at first. If you are encountering a great amount of difficulty then perhaps working with another person would be of benefit.

A last item that you should pay special attention to is the symbol ▶. This is used throughout the text to readily identify directions that you are to follow while progressing through this text.

TASK ANALYSIS

The following is a summarization, or task analysis of your progression through each chapter:

1. Take the pretest only if you have previous skills in this area and feel you already possess the performance objectives of the chapter.
2. Read/understand/memorize the contents of the text.
3. Complete the activity sheet and correct it using the answers at the end of the chapter.
4. When inaccuracies occur, restudy the text, and then recalculate any incorrect problems.
5. Repeat steps 2 through 4 for any subsequent text and activity sheets in the chapter.
6. Complete the posttest and correct it.
7. a. If all your answers are correct, proceed to the next chapter.
   b. If your answers indicate inadequacies in learning return to the appropriate (i) text and review and (ii) activity sheet(s) for more practice. Then correct the errors on the posttest. Take the chapter pretest as a second posttest, and correct it. Be sure to master this chapter before proceeding to the next.

With the preceding directions in mind, you are ready to begin this learning experience. I do hope that you find it as challenging, profitable, and enjoyable as have the previous students with whom I have worked.

2 | *Evaluation of Prerequisite Mathematics Skills*

Self-assessment Mathematics Test

OBJECTIVE

The overall purpose of this test is self-assessment of your mathematical competency. The test was specifically designed to evaluate skills necessary to learning the mathematical contents of this book.

Take this test without referring to other resources so that you can accurately assess your current mathematical abilities.

PART I: FRACTIONS

1. Add:

   (a) $\dfrac{6}{17} + \dfrac{5}{17} + \dfrac{2}{17}$

   (b) $\dfrac{1}{18} + \dfrac{1}{9} + \dfrac{1}{36} + \dfrac{1}{4}$

   (c) $2\dfrac{1}{6} + \dfrac{1}{9} + 1\dfrac{1}{3} + \dfrac{1}{5}$

2. Subtract:

   (a) $\dfrac{5}{12} - \dfrac{2}{9}$

   (b) $15\dfrac{7}{8} - 11\dfrac{3}{10}$

3. Reduce these fractions:

   (a) $\dfrac{6}{8}$ (b) $\dfrac{58}{87}$ (c) $\dfrac{21}{240}$

4. Multiply:

   (a) $\dfrac{1}{4} \times \dfrac{1}{8}$ (b) $\dfrac{2}{15} \times 10$

   (c) $\dfrac{5}{12} \times \dfrac{10}{87}$ (d) $\dfrac{1}{150} \times 3$

5. Divide:

   (a) $\dfrac{1}{32} \div \dfrac{1}{8}$

   (b) $\dfrac{\frac{1}{36}}{2}$

   (c) $\dfrac{9}{10} \div \dfrac{4}{5}$

   (d) $\dfrac{\frac{1}{120}}{\frac{1}{60}}$

6. Arrange the following fractions in ascending order, from smallest to largest:

   $\dfrac{1}{4} ; \dfrac{1}{6} ; \dfrac{1}{2} ; \dfrac{1}{8} ; \dfrac{1}{3}$

7. Arrange the following in ascending order, from smallest to largest:

   $\dfrac{5}{9} ; \dfrac{9}{10} ; \dfrac{3}{5} ; \dfrac{7}{8} ; \dfrac{2}{3}$

8. Change the following mixed numbers to improper fractions:

   (a) $152\dfrac{3}{4}$

   (b) $42\dfrac{9}{10}$

9. Change the following improper fractions to mixed numbers:

   (a) $\dfrac{35}{8}$

   (b) $\dfrac{593}{10}$

PART II: DECIMALS

10. Name the positions of the following numbers: 5.3694

11. The decimal 0.0052 is read as _____ .

12. Add:
    (a) $0.125 + 0.125$
    (b) $2.101 + 3.9 + 0.029$

13. Subtract:
    (a) $21.35 - 2.001$
    (b) $2.0 - 0.906$

14. Multiply:
    (a) 0.302×100
    (b) 0.5×0.5
    (c) 3.1×1.75
    (d) 0.25×5

15. Divide:
    (a) $3.076 \div 100$ (b) $0.5 \div 0.125$
    (c) $0.5 \div 2$ (d) $1.5 \div 0.25$

16. Place the following numbers in the correct progression from lowest to highest in value:
    5.42; 0.5205; 5.005; 50.005; 50.012

17. Place the following numbers in the correct progression from highest to lowest in value:
    0.4; 0.25; 0.125; 0.375; 0.05

PART III: CONVERSION

18. The decimal 0.005 expressed as a fraction, reduced to its lowest terms, is _____ .

19. The decimal 0.16 expressed as a fraction, reduced to its lowest terms, is _____ .

20. The fraction $\dfrac{1}{25}$ expressed as a decimal equals _____ .

21. The fraction $\dfrac{92}{6}$ expressed as a decimal equals _____ .

PART IV: PERCENTAGES

22. Express as a fraction:

    (a) 3%   (b) $\dfrac{1}{2}$%

23. Express as a percent:
    (a) $\dfrac{1}{4}$ (b) $\dfrac{2}{5}$

24. Express as a decimal:
    (a) 0.9%   (b) 100%

25. Express as a percent:
    (a) 0.07   (b) 2.25

26. Compute the following:
    (a) 50% of 150 is _____ .
    (b) 75% of 12 is _____ .
    (c) What percent of 36 is 6?
    (d) What percent of 60 is 15?

PART V: RATIOS

27. Write the following fraction-form ratios as colon-form ratios:

    (a) $\dfrac{9}{10}$ (b) $\dfrac{63}{70}$ (c) $\dfrac{\frac{1}{2}}{5}$ (d) $\dfrac{3}{4\frac{1}{5}}$

    (e) $10 \div 40$ (f) 5   (g) 75%

28. Convert the following ratios as indicated
    (a) $\dfrac{1}{4}:7$ _____ (fraction)
    (b) 4:5 _____ (decimal)
    (c) 2:3 _____ %

29. Write the numerical ratio for the following statements:
    (a) There are five patients to every nurse.
    (b) There are 10 pills to each bottle.
    (c) Five grains are in each pill.
    (d) Twenty grains are in four pills.

PART VI: PROPORTIONS

30. Write the proportions for the following statements (use x for the unknown factor):
    (a) There are five patients to every nurse. To take care of 115 patients, how many nurses are needed?
    (b) There are ten pills in each bottle. Forty-five pills are contained in how many bottles?
    (c) If 5 grains are in each pill, how many grains are in 23 pills?
    (d) If 20 grains are in four pills, how many grains are in half a pill?

31. Solve the following:
    (a) $\dfrac{x}{9} = \dfrac{4}{72}$ (b) $\dfrac{5}{x} = \dfrac{3}{15}$

    (c) $\dfrac{5}{0.9} = \dfrac{x}{0.27}$ (d) $\dfrac{\frac{1}{2}}{1} = \dfrac{\frac{1}{4}}{x}$

32. Solve the following
   (a) $2:8::5:x$
   (b) $3:x::5:8$
   (c) $0.5:x::0.125:4$
   (d) $\frac{2}{3}:x::\frac{3}{4}:\frac{9}{10}$

PART VII: PROBLEM SOLVING

33. If each basket contains 16 apples, how many baskets would you buy to obtain 96 apples?

34. It takes 5 tablespoons of ground coffee to make 6 cups of coffee. How many tablespoons of ground coffee would you need to make 300 cups of coffee?

35. In a group the ratio of men to women is $5:8$. The total group is 260. How many women are in this group?

36. Each book weighs 1.25 lb. The bookshelf has a capacity of 14 lb. How many books can be safely placed on it?

37. One bottle has 30 pills in it. To have 105 pills, how many bottles must you have?

38. You must have 1 teaspoon of fluid available for each 5 lb a person weighs. How much should you have for a 115-lb person?

39. Each tablet has 7 units in it. To administer 17.5 units, how many tablets should you give?

▶ Upon completion of this test, compare your answers with the answer sheet that follows. If you have incorrect answers, take special time and care to review the areas that were difficult for you. These difficult areas may interfere with your progress throughout the book. Rather than beginning Part II, Mastering Drug Dosage Calculations, you are advised to first complete the mathematics review section (Chapter 3) of this book.

Answers for Chapter 2

PART I

1. (a) $\dfrac{13}{17}$ (b) $\dfrac{4}{9}$ (c) $3\dfrac{73}{90}$

2. (a) $\dfrac{7}{36}$ (b) $4\dfrac{23}{40}$

3. (a) $\dfrac{3}{4}$ (b) $\dfrac{2}{3}$ (c) $\dfrac{7}{80}$

4. (a) $\dfrac{1}{32}$ (b) $1\dfrac{1}{3}$ (c) $\dfrac{25}{522}$ (d) $\dfrac{1}{50}$

5. (a) $\dfrac{1}{4}$ (b) $\dfrac{1}{72}$ (c) $1\dfrac{1}{8}$ (d) $\dfrac{1}{2}$

6. $\dfrac{1}{8}; \dfrac{1}{6}; \dfrac{1}{4}; \dfrac{1}{3}; \dfrac{1}{2}$

7. $\dfrac{5}{9}; \dfrac{3}{5}; \dfrac{2}{3}; \dfrac{7}{8}; \dfrac{9}{10}$

8. (a) $\dfrac{611}{4}$ (b) $\dfrac{429}{10}$ 9. (a) $4\dfrac{3}{8}$ (b) $59\dfrac{3}{10}$

PART II

10. 5 = units, 3 = tenths, 6 = hundredths, 9 = thousandths, 4 = ten-thousandths

11. Fifty-two ten-thousandths

12. (a) 0.25   (b) 6.03

13. (a) 19.349   (b) 1.094

14. (a) 30.2   (b) 0.25   (c) 5.425   (d) 1.25

15. (a) 0.03076   (b) 4   (c) 0.25   (d) 6

16. 0.5205; 5.005; 5.42; 50.005; 50.012

17. 0.4; 0.375; 0.25; 0.125; 0.05

PART III

18. $\dfrac{1}{200}$ 19. $\dfrac{4}{25}$ 20. 0.04   21. 15.33

PART IV

22. (a) $\dfrac{3}{100}$ (b) $\dfrac{\frac{1}{2}}{100}$ or $\dfrac{1}{200}$

23. (a) 25%   (b) 40%
24. (a) 0.009   (b) 1.0
25. (a) 7%   (b) 225%

26. (a) 75   (b) 9   (c) $16\dfrac{2}{3}\%$ (d) 25%

PART V

27. (a) 9:10   (b) 63:70 or 9:10   (c) $\dfrac{1}{2}:5$ (d) $3:4\dfrac{1}{5}$
    (e) 10:40 or 1:4   (f) 5:1   (g) 75:100 or 3:4

28. (a) $\dfrac{\frac{1}{4}}{7}$ (b) 0.8   (c) $66\dfrac{2}{3}$

29. (a) 5:1 or $\dfrac{5}{1}$ (b) 10:1 or $\dfrac{10}{1}$
    (c) 5:1 or $\dfrac{5}{1}$ (d) 20:4 or 5:1 or $\dfrac{20}{4}$ or $\dfrac{5}{1}$

PART VI

30. (a) $\dfrac{5 \text{ patients}}{1 \text{ nurse}} = \dfrac{115 \text{ patients}}{x \text{ nurses}}$

    (b) $\dfrac{10 \text{ pills}}{1 \text{ bottle}} = \dfrac{45 \text{ pills}}{x \text{ bottles}}$

    (c) $\dfrac{5 \text{ gr}}{1 \text{ pill}} = \dfrac{x \text{ gr}}{23 \text{ pills}}$

    (d) $\dfrac{20 \text{ gr}}{4 \text{ pills}} = \dfrac{x \text{ gr}}{\frac{1}{2} \text{ pill}}$

31. (a) $\frac{1}{2}$ (b) 25   (c) 1.5   (d) $\frac{1}{2}$

32. (a) 20   (b) $4\frac{4}{5}$ or 4.8   (c) 16   (d) $\frac{4}{5}$

PART VII

33. 6   34. 250   35. 160   36. 11   37. $3\frac{1}{2}$ 38. 23

39. $2\frac{1}{2}$ or 2.5

3 | *Basic/General Mathematics Review*

FRACTIONS

General Information

A **fraction** is a part, portion, or section of a whole (entity). When used numerically it refers to taking a whole number and dividing it into equal parts, portions, or sections. An example expressed numerically would be:

$$3/4 \text{ or } \frac{3}{4}$$

(depending on how one chooses to write it). In a fraction the number that lies to the right of the diagonal line or below the horizontal line is called the **denominator**. The denominator tells you how many parts, portions, or sections that whole number is divided into. In this example the whole is divided into 4 equal parts. The denominator is also called the **divisor**. The divisor tells you how many parts, portions, or sections a whole should be divided into.

The number that lies to the left of the diagonal line or above the horizontal line is called the **numerator**. It represents a certain number or amount of parts, portions, or sections. For example, in the above case the number 3 indicates that you are working with 3 of the total 4 parts. If it were a pie, you would have 3 pieces of the total number of pieces that you cut it into.

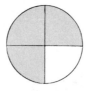

3 Sections = *Numerator*   Total 4 sections = *Denominator*

The numerator is called the **dividend** and tells you how many parts of that whole you are working with.

Terminology

A **proper fraction** is a fraction in which the value of the numerator is less than the denominator.

Example

$$\frac{2}{3}, \frac{3}{7}, \text{ or } \frac{4}{9}.$$

An **improper fraction** is a fraction in which the value of the numerator is greater than the denominator.

Example

$$\frac{3}{2}, \frac{7}{3}, \text{ or } \frac{9}{4}.$$

A **complex fraction** is a fraction that is composed of fractions or fractions and whole numbers.

Example

$$\frac{\frac{2}{3}}{\frac{4}{9}} \text{ or } \frac{\frac{2}{3}}{4}.$$

A **mixed number** is a numerical value that contains a whole number followed by a fractional amount.

Example

$$5\frac{15}{22} \text{ or } 10\frac{5}{8}.$$

Addition of Fractions with Denominators All Equal

To add fractions you must make the denominators the same.

Example

$$\frac{1}{17} + \frac{2}{17} + \frac{9}{17}.$$

To add these fractions merely add the numerators and write this numerical value over the denominator. What you have done is found the total number of parts (numerator) of the whole (denominator) you are working with. *Answer: 12/17*

Practice Problems

1. $\frac{1}{11} + \frac{3}{11} + \frac{4}{11} =$

2. $\frac{2}{13} + \frac{1}{13} + \frac{5}{13} =$

3. $\frac{7}{19} + \frac{10}{19} + \frac{1}{19} =$

Addition of Fractions with Varied Denominator Values

Step 1: Find the lowest common denominator. If fractions need to be added and their denominators are of different values, you must find what is called the lowest or least common denominator (LCD) before you can add them. The **lowest common denominator** is the smallest number into which each of the denominators can be divided evenly. A good starting point is to see if all the denominators can be evenly divided into the denominator of the highest value. If this is not possible, proceed to find the smallest multiple of the largest denominator in the problem you are working on that each of the smaller denominators can be divided into evenly.

Example

$$\frac{1}{2} + \frac{3}{16} + \frac{1}{32}.$$

In this example, 2 and 16 can be divided evenly into 32. Therefore 32 is considered the least common denominator for this problem. This means that the whole (the denominator) that is common to all of these fractions is divided into 32 sections.

Step 2: Using 32 (the LCD) as the denominator of all the fractions find the numerator that will make the new fraction (with 32 in the denominator) equivalent to the original fraction:

$$\frac{1}{2} = \frac{?}{32}$$

To find the new numerator you divide the LCD by the denominator of the original fraction and then multiply the result by the numerator of the original fraction. In this problem 32 divided by 2 equals 16, and 16 multiplied by the original numerator (1) is equal to 16; therefore

$$\text{the new numerator is 16, i.e., } \frac{1}{2} = \frac{16}{32}.$$

$$\frac{3}{16} = \frac{?}{32}$$

In this problem 32 divided by 16 equals 2, and 2 multiplied by the original numerator (3) equals 6; therefore

$$\text{the new numerator is 6, i.e., } \frac{3}{16} = \frac{6}{32}.$$

Step 3: After all fractions have a common denominator the numerators are added:

$$\frac{16}{32} + \frac{6}{32} + \frac{1}{32} = \frac{23}{32}$$

Example

$$\frac{1}{3} + \frac{1}{13}.$$

Step 1: Find the lowest common denominator.
Note: 3 does not divide into 13.
Now see if 3 divides into a multiple of 13: $13 \times 2 = 26$.
No. $13 \times 3 = 39$. Yes. Therefore, $39 = \text{LCD}$.

Step 2: Convert the fractions as was done in the previous example.

$$\frac{1}{3} = \frac{?}{39}$$

In this problem 39 divided by 3 is equal to 13 and 13 multiplied by the original numerator (1) is equal to 13, so

$$\text{the new numerator is 13, i.e., } \frac{1}{3} = \frac{13}{39}.$$

$$\frac{1}{13} = \frac{?}{39}$$

In this problem 39 divided by 13 equals 3, and 3 multiplied by the original numerator (1) equals 3, so

$$\text{the new numerator is 3, i.e., } \frac{1}{13} = \frac{3}{39}.$$

Step 3: After all fractions have been changed and have a common denominator, the numerators are added:

$$\frac{1}{3} + \frac{1}{13} = \frac{13}{39} + \frac{3}{39}$$

$$= \frac{16}{39}$$

Practice Problems

4. $\dfrac{1}{19} + \dfrac{5}{38} =$

5. $\dfrac{1}{2} + \dfrac{3}{7} =$

6. $\dfrac{1}{3} + \dfrac{1}{15} + \dfrac{1}{45} =$

7. $\dfrac{1}{3} + \dfrac{2}{7} =$

Addition of Fractions with Mixed Numbers

Step 1: Add the fractions (remember to find the LCD) when necessary).

Step 2: Add the whole numbers.

Step 3: Add the sums together.

Example

$1\dfrac{1}{8} + 3\dfrac{3}{16}$.

Add fractions: $\dfrac{1}{8} + \dfrac{3}{16} = \dfrac{2}{16} + \dfrac{3}{16} = \dfrac{5}{16}$ (step 1).

Add whole numbers: $1 + 3 = 4$ (step 2).

Answer: $4 + \dfrac{5}{16} = 4\dfrac{5}{16}$ (step 3).

Practice Problems

8. $2\dfrac{1}{2} + 1\dfrac{1}{10} + \dfrac{1}{10} =$

9. $3\dfrac{1}{3} + \dfrac{2}{5} =$

10. $4\dfrac{3}{4} + \dfrac{1}{12} =$

Subtraction of Fractions with Equal Denominators

As in addition, to subtract fractions you must make the denominators the same. If they are not the same, first find the LCD and then subtract the numerators.

Example

$$\frac{7}{13} - \frac{5}{13} = \frac{2}{13}.$$

$$\frac{5}{6} - \frac{5}{12} = \frac{10}{12} - \frac{5}{12} = \frac{5}{12}.$$

Practice Problems

11. $\dfrac{7}{13} - \dfrac{4}{13} =$

12. $\dfrac{5}{9} - \dfrac{3}{18} =$

13. $\dfrac{13}{19} - \dfrac{10}{19} =$

14. $\dfrac{2}{3} - \dfrac{5}{18} =$

15. $\dfrac{11}{21} - \dfrac{5}{21} =$

16. $\dfrac{2}{7} - \dfrac{1}{21} =$

Subtraction of Fractions with Whole Numbers and Small Fractions

When fractions are to be subtracted from whole numbers and when the top fraction is smaller in value one must borrow a whole number from the number next to that fraction before subtraction can occur. As in the previous examples, the denominators must be the same or the LCD must be found before proceeding. Subtract the whole numbers, and subtract fractions.

Example

$$2\frac{7}{11} - 1\frac{3}{11}.$$

Subtract whole numbers: $2 - 1 = 1$.

Subtract fractions: $\dfrac{7}{11} - \dfrac{3}{11} = \dfrac{4}{11}.$

Answer:
$$2\frac{7}{11}$$
$$-1\frac{3}{11}$$
$$\overline{\quad 1\frac{4}{11}\quad}$$

Example

$$3\frac{3}{7}$$
$$-1\frac{6}{7}$$
$$\overline{\qquad\qquad}$$

Borrowing 1: $\quad 2\left(\dfrac{7}{7}+\dfrac{3}{7}\right)$ $\qquad$ Answer: $\quad 2\dfrac{10}{7}$

$$-1\frac{6}{7}$$
$$\overline{\qquad\qquad\qquad}$$

$$-1\frac{6}{7}$$
$$\overline{\qquad\quad 1\frac{4}{7}}$$

In order to borrow one, you make a fraction in which the numerator is the same number as the denominator. In this example, 7/7 = 1. Other examples are

$$\frac{9}{9}=1,\quad \frac{10}{10}=1,\quad \frac{11}{11}=1.$$

You now have the

$$\frac{7}{7}\text{ plus the original }\frac{3}{7}\text{, a total of }\frac{10}{7},$$

in the fraction column, and can do the subtraction.

Practice Problems

17. $\quad 4\dfrac{5}{9}$

$$-2\frac{1}{9}$$
$$\overline{\qquad\qquad}$$

18. $\quad 6\dfrac{7}{13}$

$$-2\frac{5}{13}$$
$$\overline{\qquad\qquad}$$

19. $5\dfrac{1}{2}$

$-2\dfrac{3}{4}$

_____

20. $7\dfrac{2}{21}$

$-5\dfrac{2}{7}$

_____

Reducing Fractions to Their Lowest Terms

Fractions are usually written in their lowest terms. One does this by dividing both the numerator and the denominator by the largest number that will divide evenly into both of them. Performing the *same* mathematical process to each (the numerator and denominator) will not change the value of the fraction. You should always check a fractional amount and reduce it to its lowest terms. This process is also called **simplifying** the fraction.

Example

Simplify $\dfrac{14}{21}$.

Both numerator and denominator can be divided by 7. Therefore

$$\frac{14}{21} = \frac{2}{3} .$$

Practice Problems

Reduce to the lowest terms.

21. $\dfrac{9}{18}$

22. $\dfrac{21}{42}$

23. $\dfrac{4}{6}$

24. $\dfrac{15}{45}$

25. $\dfrac{12}{48}$

Improper Fractions

An **improper fraction** is a term used when the numerator has a higher value than the denominator. If this occurs at the end of a problem, it is best to write this as a whole number plus a fraction. Do this by dividing the denominator into the numerator—this gives you the whole number. Then the number that is left over becomes the numerator of the fractional amount left over.

Example

$\frac{8}{6}$.

6 divided into 8 is 1 with 2 left over and 2 becomes the numerator of the fractional amount. Therefore,

$$\frac{8}{6} = 1\frac{2}{6} = 1\frac{1}{3}.$$

Remember here that fractions should be reduced to their lowest terms.

Practice Problems

Write the following fractions as mixed numbers:

26. $\frac{21}{8}$

27. $\frac{18}{7}$

28. $\frac{9}{6}$

29. $\frac{10}{8}$

30. $\frac{15}{6}$

Changing Numbers to Improper Fractions

There are occasions when a mixed number must be changed to an improper fraction in order to solve a problem. To do this, perform the following steps:

Step 1: Multiply the whole number by the denominator of the fraction.

Step 2: Add the product obtained in step 1 to the numerical value of the numerator of the fraction.

Step 3: Use the sum obtained in step 2 as the numerator of the improper fraction. The denominator of this fraction remains the original number.

Example

Write $3\frac{7}{9}$ as an improper fraction.

Step 1: $3 \times 9 = 27$.

Step 2: $27 + 7 = 34$.

Step 3: $\frac{34}{9}$.

Practice Problems

Write the following mixed numbers as improper fractions:

31. $2\frac{5}{6}$

32. $5\frac{3}{10}$

33. $6\frac{2}{9}$

34. $4\frac{5}{8}$

35. $1\frac{5}{9}$

Multiplication of Fractions

Fractions are multiplied by multiplying the two numerators to obtain the numerator of the answer and then multiplying the two denominators to obtain the denominator of the answer.

Example

$\frac{3}{5} \times \frac{1}{2}$.

$3 \times 1 = 3$ (to find numerator)

$5 \times 2 = 10$ (to find denominator)

$\frac{3}{5} \times \frac{1}{2} = \frac{3}{10}$

Be sure to reduce your answer to lowest terms, if necessary.

Practice Problems

36. $\frac{3}{4} \times \frac{1}{2} =$

37. $\dfrac{2}{8} \times \dfrac{1}{4} =$

38. $\dfrac{1}{3} \times \dfrac{7}{10} =$

39. $\dfrac{2}{7} \times \dfrac{1}{9} =$

40. $\dfrac{3}{12} \times \dfrac{1}{3} =$

Cancellation Used During Multiplication

Cancellation is a process that can be used when multiplying fractions. It occurs when the numerator and denominator of fractions to be multiplied are divided by the same number; that number should always be the largest number to divide evenly.

Example

$$\frac{2}{15} \times \frac{5}{8} = \frac{\overset{1}{\cancel{2}}}{15} \times \frac{5}{\underset{4}{\cancel{8}}}$$

$$= \frac{1}{\underset{3}{\cancel{15}}} \times \frac{\overset{1}{\cancel{5}}}{4}$$

$$= \frac{1}{3} \times \frac{1}{4}$$

$$= \frac{1}{12}$$

Practice Problems

Perform cancellation:

41. $\dfrac{2}{5} \times \dfrac{5}{7}$

42. $\dfrac{1}{6} \times \dfrac{3}{8}$

43. $\dfrac{1}{2} \times \dfrac{8}{17}$

44. $\dfrac{1}{3} \times \dfrac{3}{7} \times \dfrac{7}{9}$

45. $\dfrac{2}{3} \times \dfrac{6}{11} \times \dfrac{22}{31}$

Multiplication of Fractions and Whole Numbers

Multiplication of fractions and whole numbers is basically the same as multiplication of fractions. The whole number is simply converted into a fraction, that is, 4 = 4/1, 5 = 5/1, etc. (The denominator for a whole number is understood to be 1; if, at the end of a problem, the answer were 4/1, we would convert it to the whole number 4.)

Example

$$\frac{1}{3} \times 4 = \frac{1}{3} \times \frac{4}{1} = \frac{4}{3} = 1\frac{1}{3}$$

Practice Problems

46. $\dfrac{1}{2} \times 9 =$

47. $\dfrac{1}{3} \times 6 =$

48. $\dfrac{2}{15} \times 5 =$

49. $\dfrac{1}{4} \times 5 =$

50. $\dfrac{1}{9} \times 3 =$

Multiplication of Fractions by Mixed Numbers or Mixed Numbers by Mixed Numbers

When multiplication involves mixed numbers, the mixed numbers should be changed to improper fractions and then multiplied.

Example

$$4\frac{1}{8} \times 1\frac{1}{3} = \frac{33}{8} \times \frac{4}{3}$$

$$= \frac{\overset{11}{\cancel{33}}}{\underset{2}{\cancel{8}}} \times \frac{\overset{1}{\cancel{4}}}{\underset{1}{\cancel{3}}} = \frac{11}{2} = 5\frac{1}{2}$$

Practice Problems

51. $\dfrac{1}{2} \times 2\dfrac{1}{4} =$

52. $\dfrac{2}{3} \times 1\dfrac{1}{2} =$

53. $\dfrac{3}{7} \times 3\dfrac{1}{3} =$

54. $\dfrac{1}{5} \times 2\dfrac{1}{6} =$

55. $1\dfrac{1}{7} \times 1\dfrac{1}{8} =$

Division of Fractions

The division of fractions is easy if you remember to *invert* the number that *follows* the *division sign*. After this is done, the numbers are multiplied. Remember that all the rules and guidelines discussed for multiplication will pertain, for example, cancellation, changing mixed numbers to improper fractions before you solve, reducing fractional answers, and leaving answers as mixed numbers (not improper fractions) when they occur.

Example

$$\dfrac{1}{2} \div \dfrac{1}{4}$$

$$= \dfrac{1}{2} \times \dfrac{4}{1} \leftarrow \text{Number following division sign inverted}$$

$$= \dfrac{1}{\cancel{2}} \times \dfrac{\cancel{4}^{2}}{1}$$

$$= \dfrac{2}{1} = 2$$

$$\dfrac{2}{3} \div 9$$

$$= \dfrac{2}{3} \times \dfrac{1}{9} \leftarrow \begin{array}{l} \text{Inversion—remember in fractions a whole} \\ \text{number has the number 1 as its denominator.} \end{array}$$

$$= \dfrac{2}{27}$$

Practice Problems

56. $\dfrac{4}{7} \div \dfrac{3}{14} =$

57. $\dfrac{4}{9} \div 3\dfrac{1}{3} =$

58. $\dfrac{1}{2} \div \dfrac{1}{8} =$

59. $4\dfrac{1}{8} \div 1\dfrac{1}{2} =$

60. $5\dfrac{1}{4} \div 2 =$

Multiplication of Complex Fractions

A **complex fraction** is a fraction in which the numerator or denominator (or both) is also a fraction, e.g.,

$$\dfrac{\dfrac{1}{3}}{\dfrac{1}{6}} .$$

A problem containing complex fractions is easy to solve if you proceed one step at a time.

Example

$$\dfrac{\dfrac{1}{3}}{\dfrac{1}{6}} \times \dfrac{\dfrac{1}{6}}{2} .$$

Step 1: Perform multiplication just as you would for regular fractions. Multiply the numerators, then denominators

$$\dfrac{\dfrac{1}{3}}{\dfrac{1}{6}} \times \dfrac{\dfrac{1}{6}}{2} = \dfrac{\dfrac{1}{18}}{\dfrac{1}{3}}$$

Step 2: Solve or re-express your answer. The above answer

$$\dfrac{\dfrac{1}{18}}{\dfrac{1}{3}} \text{ means } \dfrac{1}{18} \text{ is divided by } \dfrac{1}{3} .$$

To do this, solve as any fractional division:

$$\frac{1}{18} \div \frac{1}{3} = \frac{1}{18} \times \frac{3}{1}$$ (Remember you must invert and multiply to solve.)

$$= \frac{1}{\cancelto{}{18}_{6}} \times \frac{\cancelto{1}{3}}{1} = \frac{1}{6}$$ (the answer to the problem)

Practice Problems

61. $\dfrac{\frac{1}{2}}{\frac{1}{4}} \times \dfrac{\frac{4}{1}}{\frac{1}{8}} =$

62. $\dfrac{\frac{1}{3}}{\frac{1}{9}} \times \dfrac{\frac{1}{3}}{\frac{1}{9}} =$

63. $\dfrac{\frac{1}{5}}{\frac{5}{1}} \times \dfrac{\frac{1}{2}}{\frac{2}{1}} =$

64. $\dfrac{\frac{1}{7}}{\frac{3}{1}} \times \dfrac{\frac{1}{3}}{\frac{7}{1}} =$

65. $\dfrac{\frac{1}{6}}{\frac{1}{3}} \times \dfrac{\frac{6}{1}}{\frac{3}{1}} =$

Values of Fractions

To evaluate the value of a list of fractions with varied denominators and then place them in either ascending or descending order of value is relatively easy. What should be done first is to find the lowest common denominator (as practiced earlier—if you do not remember, review it). Once each fraction is expressed in terms of that LCD, it is easy to compare their value.

Example

Evaluate $\dfrac{2}{7}, \dfrac{1}{2}, \dfrac{3}{14}$.

The lowest common denominator is 14.

$$\frac{2}{7} = \frac{4}{14} \quad \text{(second highest value)}$$

$$\frac{1}{2} = \frac{7}{14} \quad \text{(highest value)}$$

$$\frac{3}{14} = \frac{3}{14} \quad \text{(lowest value)}$$

Practice Problems

List in descending order:

66. $\dfrac{1}{3}, \dfrac{1}{2}, \dfrac{1}{4}, \dfrac{1}{8}$

67. $\dfrac{2}{5}, \dfrac{3}{10}, \dfrac{1}{100}, \dfrac{6}{25}$

68. $\dfrac{1}{16}, \dfrac{1}{4}, \dfrac{3}{32}, \dfrac{3}{8}$

69. $\dfrac{7}{18}, \dfrac{1}{6}, \dfrac{1}{3}, \dfrac{1}{2}$

DECIMALS

General Information

Decimals are another means of expressing a fractional amount. They are, however, written or expressed differently. A decimal point placed *before* a number indicates that a fractional amount follows. Fractions have a numerator and a denominator: one can think of decimals as fractions also. The numerator in a decimal is the number that *follows* the decimal point, for example, in 1.5, the 5 is the numerator. The number falling before the decimal point is a whole number. One could equate this to a mixed number.

The denominators used in decimals are consistent; they are multiples of ten. The denominator can be readily understood or stated knowing the position of a number or numbers that follow the decimal point, for the position name indicates the numerical value of the understood denominator.

Example

5.12345. The names of the positions are as follows:

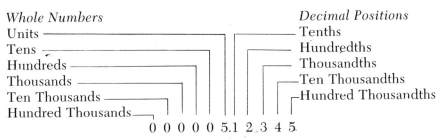

The denominator taken to read this number (5.12345) is hundred thousandths. You always use the highest position. Do not read each number/position separately. This number would be read five (whole numbers are always read first) and (the "and" indicates the decimal point) twelve thousand three hundred forth-five hundred thousandths. Five and twelve thousand three hundred forty-five hundred thousandths written as a mixed number would be

$$5\frac{12,345}{100,000}.$$

The zero used in decimals is very meaningful. If it occurs before a number it is very important in that it indicates a position and relates the proper value of that number. For example, 2.01 is two and one hundredths; if the zero were not there (i.e., 2.1), the decimal value would be one tenth. Now if the zero occurs at the end of a decimal number, it has no value and can be eliminated (which is not true of a zero used with whole numbers). The zero in 2.10 can be eliminated since

$$2\frac{10}{100} \text{ is the same value as } 2\frac{1}{10}$$

and therefore 2.10 = 2.1.

Practice Problems

Write how you would read the following decimal values and then write them as a fraction or mixed number:

70. 100,000.3
71. 15,000.27
72. 2,000.149
73. 500.0534
74. 7.023
75. 0.03
76. 15.00015

Write out the following as decimals and then as fractions:
77. Five and three hundred thousandths
78. Two hundred twenty-seven ten thousandths
79. Fifteen and five hundredths
80. Six and six tenths
81. Seven thousandths
82. Nine and nine ten thousandths
83. One hundred twenty-three thousandths

Write the following fractions as decimals and then write them as they would be read aloud:

84. $100,000 \frac{7}{10}$

85. $1 \frac{87}{100}$

86. $13 \frac{527}{1000}$

87. $\frac{37}{10,000}$

88. $\frac{127}{100,000}$

What is the best way to write the following as decimals?

89. $\frac{3}{100}$

90. $\frac{20}{100}$

91. $\frac{107}{1000}$

92. $\frac{5}{10}$

93. $\frac{50}{100}$

94. $5 \frac{100}{1000}$

95. $5 \frac{230}{1000}$

Addition and Subtraction of Decimals

To add and subtract decimals is relatively easy. It is basically done as one adds and subtracts whole numbers. What must be remembered is to align the decimal points of the various numbers so that the positions of the numbers are kept in order before beginning to add or subtract.

Example

6 + 12.03 + 5.125 + 0.0004 + 3.7 + 100.02374.

$$
\begin{array}{r}
6. \\
12.03 \\
5.125 \\
0.0004 \\
3.7 \\
\underline{100.02374} \\
126.87914
\end{array}
$$

10.327 − 5.6.

$$
\begin{array}{r}
10.327 \\
\underline{-5.6} \\
4.727
\end{array}
$$

Practice Problems

96. 5.3 + 12.713 + 909.0071 + 0.02 =

97. 3.01 + 0.4834 + 7.7 + 8.707 =

98. 10.5 + 15.15 + 7 + 3.101 =

99. 1.125 + 2.03 + 5 + 3.0006 =

100. 8.03 + 4.4 + 10.010 + 0.8281 =

101. 3.785 − 2.705 =

102. 10.36 − 5.3 =

103. 15.888 − 5.488 =

104. 3.468 − 0.312 =

105. 101.321 − 1.307 =

Multiplication of Decimals

The multiplication of decimals is done in the same manner as multiplication of whole numbers, with the exception that the decimal point must be placed accurately in the product (the answer obtained after multiplying the two numbers). To assure the proper placement of the decimal point do not attempt to do this until the product is obtained.

To determine the decimal point's placement, *first* count the total number of places to the right of the decimal points of the numbers being multiplied. (In example A below, this is 4; in example B it is 3.) After you have obtained this number, count that many positions in the product starting from right to left (see below). Then place the decimal point before the last position counted.

Example A

$$
\begin{array}{r}
3.71 \\
\times 0.43 \\
\hline
1113 \\
1484 \\
\hline
1.5953
\end{array}
$$

3.71 ← 2 places
×0.43 ← 2 places
1113   (total 4 places)
1484
1.5953   4 places

4 3 2 1   Answer = 1.5953

Example B

0.006 ← 3 places
×5
0.030   3 places

3 2 1   Answer = 0.03

When your product seems to have a decreased number of places (as in example B), be sure that zeros are placed in the answer until placement of the decimal point occurs. Then if a zero is at the end, as in example B, it can be eliminated.

Practice Problems

106. $14.2 \times 0.36 =$
107. $4 \times 0.07 =$
108. $3.12 \times 0.12 =$
109. $7 \times 0.7 =$
110. $0.5 \times 0.5 =$
111. $0.25 \times 0.25 =$

Division of Decimals

Division of decimals is done in much the same way as division of whole numbers. The difference lies in knowing what to do with the decimal point. To discuss and understand this, terminology of a typical division set up should be remembered:

$$\text{divisor } \overline{)\text{dividend}}^{\text{quotient}}$$

When the divisor is a whole number, then the decimal point in the answer (quotient) should be placed immediately above the decimal point in the dividend, for example, $5\overline{)3.525}$. It is helpful to place it there before the division calculation takes place.

When the divisor contains a decimal, move the decimal the number of places to the right necessary to make it a whole number. After this, move the decimal point in the dividend an equal number of places to the right. Then place a decimal point in the quotient space exactly above the one in the dividend.

Example

$$
5\overline{)3.525} = 5\overline{)3.525} = \begin{array}{r} 0.705 \\ 5\overline{)3.525} \\ \underline{35} \\ 002 \\ \underline{0} \\ 25 \\ \underline{25} \end{array}
$$

$$
3.25\overline{)4.1275} = 3.25\,\overline{)4.1275} = \begin{array}{r} 1.27 \\ 325\overline{)412.75} \\ \underline{325} \\ 877 \\ \underline{650} \\ 2275 \\ \underline{2275} \end{array}
$$

If there is an inadequate number of places to move the decimal point, add zeros.

Example

$$
0.25\,\overline{)2} = 0.25\overline{)2.00}
$$

Practice Problems

112. $3.1\overline{)9.362} =$

113. $5\overline{)5.25} =$

114. $0.5\overline{)0.5} =$

115. $0.125\overline{)0.125} =$

116. $4.3\overline{)8.686} =$

Changing Fractions to Decimals

To change a fraction to a decimal, divide the denominator into the numerator.

Example

What is $\dfrac{3}{4}$ as a decimal?

$$
\begin{array}{r}
0.75 \\
4\overline{)3.00} \\
\underline{28} \\
20 \\
\underline{20}
\end{array}
$$

Practice Problems

Change the following fractions into decimals:

117. $\dfrac{1}{3} =$

118. $\dfrac{125}{1000} =$

119. $\dfrac{1}{16} =$

120. $\dfrac{3}{50} =$

121. $\dfrac{2}{25} =$

Values of Decimals

To determine the respective values of a group of decimals, compare the numbers in the position immediately to the right of the decimal point— the larger number is the larger value (e.g., 9.819 is larger than 9.091). If the numbers in the position just right of the decimal point are equal, move one position further to the right and compare these numbers (e.g., 9.89 is larger than 9.85). Lastly, if one decimal has more numbers to the right of the decimal point than the other decimal, you can add a zero to the rightmost position of the decimal with fewer places (e.g., 9.89 is the same number as 9.890 and is smaller than 9.895).

Practice Problems

Place the following in descending order:
122. 0.75, 0.08, 0.0109, 0.425, 0.275
123. 0.45, 0.052, 0.325, 0.8, 1.0
124. 0.54, 0.054, 0.0054, 0.00054
125. 0.33, 0.25, 0.75, 0.66
126. 0.125, 0.25, 0.5, 0.05

Movement of the Decimal Point

Because each position in decimals represents a multiple of ten, multiplication and division can be easily accomplished by the movement of the decimal point. Movement of the decimal point to the right is for multiplication; to the left division. Each position you move is for a multiple of ten, therefore:

a. Movement of decimal point
    one place to the right $= \times$ 10 (multiplying it by 10).
    Movement of decimal point
    two places to the right $= \times$ 100 (multiplying it by 100).
    Movement of decimal point
    three places to the right $= \times$ 1000 (multiplying it by 1000).
    Movement of decimal point
    four places to the right $= \times$ 10,000 (multiplying it by 10,000).

b. Movement of decimal point
    one place to the left $= \div$ 10 (dividing by 10).
    Movement of decimal point
    two places to the left $= \div$ 100 (dividing by 100).
    Movement of decimal point
    three places to the left $= \div$ 1000 (dividing by 1000).
    Movement of decimal point
    four places to the left $= \div$ 10,000 (dividing by 10,000).

Practice Problems

Indicate the movement of the decimal point for the following problems:

127. $6.3 \times 100 =$
128. $35.35 \div 100 =$
129. $3.75 \times 10 =$
130. $3.75 \div 10 =$
131. $15.957 \times 1000 =$
132. $15.957 \div 1000 =$
133. $33 \div 100 =$
134. $33 \times 100 =$

PERCENTAGES

General Information

The term percent refers to parts of a whole (which is 100 for percents), or parts per hundred, and is represented by the symbol %. When we talk about 30% we mean 30 parts of the whole 100%. Once again, like fractions and decimals, a percent is part of a whole.

Expressed as a fraction, a percent (%) always has a denominator of 100 and a numerator equal to the number in front of the % symbol.

Example

$$5\% = \frac{5}{100} = \frac{1}{20}.$$

To express a percent as a decimal, remember that percent means division by 100; with decimals, division by 100 is accomplished by moving the decimal point two places to the left.

Example

$$50\% = 50. = 0.50 = 0.5$$

If you are unable to move two places to the left because the percent is less than 10 (e.g. 5%), you add a zero to the left of the number.

Example

$$5\% = 05. = .05 \text{ or } 0.05.$$

Practice Problems

Change the following percents to fractions and decimals:
135. 13% =
136. 30% =
137. 25% =
138. 1.0% =
139. 15% =

Calculating the % of a Number

To perform this task change the percent to either a fraction or a decimal and then multiply the number by it.

Example

A solution contains 5% of a specific substance and the total volume is 1000 cc. What is the quantity of the specific substance?

Change the % to a fraction or a decimal:

$$5\% = \frac{5}{100} = \frac{1}{20} \quad \text{or} \quad 5\% = 0.05$$

Then multiply the number by the above fraction or decimal:

$$\overset{50}{\cancel{1000}} \times \frac{1}{\underset{1}{\cancel{20}}} = 50 \text{ cc} \quad \text{or} \quad \begin{array}{r} 1000 \\ \times\ 0.05 \\ \hline 50.00 \text{ cc} \end{array}$$

Example

A solution must total 100 cc and 10% of it must be of a specific substance. How much volume of a specific substance must be present in this solution?

Change the % to a decimal or a fraction

$$10\% = 10. = 0.1 \quad \text{or} \quad 10\% = \frac{10}{100} = \frac{1}{10}$$

Multiply the number by the above decimal or fraction

$$
\begin{array}{c}
100 \text{ cc} \\
\underline{\times 0.1} \\
10.0 \text{ cc} = 10 \text{ cc}
\end{array}
\quad \text{or} \quad
100 \times \frac{1}{10} = \overset{10}{\cancel{100}} \times \frac{1}{\cancel{10}} \\
$$

$$= 10 \text{ cc}$$

Practice Problems

140. 7% of 1000 =
141. 6% of 120 =
142. 5% of 500 =
143. 0.9% of 1000 =
144. 2.5% of 500 =

Changing a Fraction or Decimal to a Percent

If the number stated is a fraction, change the fraction to a decimal and then multiply it by 100. If the number is a decimal, you need only to multiply by 100.

Example

$$\frac{1}{25} = \text{_____} \%.$$

Change the fraction to a decimal (divide the numerator by the denominator):

$$
\begin{array}{r}
.04 \\
25\overline{)1.00} \\
\underline{100}
\end{array}
$$

Then multiply by 100:

$$0.04 \times 100 = 0.04 = 4\%$$

Practice Problems

145. $\dfrac{1}{20}$ = _____ %

146. $\dfrac{1}{10}$ = _____ %

147. $\dfrac{3}{4}$ = _____ %

148. $\dfrac{4}{5}$ = _____ %

149. $\dfrac{9}{10}$ = _____ %

150. 0.6 = _____ %

151. 0.09 = _____ %

RATIOS

A ratio is a numerical expression that shows the relationship between two quantities. Suppose we were discussing a solution that was composed of 1 part of an active ingredient and 6 parts of an inert ingredient. If we wanted to represent the relationship of these two quantities numerically we could write

$\dfrac{1}{6}$ (just as we previously wrote a fraction) or 1:6.

The / and the : both represent division signs.

Example

2 parts of an entire 7 part solution is a drug. Represent this as a ratio.
Answer: $\dfrac{2}{7}$ or 2:7.

Practice Problems

152. 7 parts of a pure drug solution per 13 parts water
153. 1 part tin per 6 parts zinc
154. 5 parts medicated solution per 7 parts NS (normal saline)
155. 4 parts item 1 per 9 parts item 2

PROPORTIONS

A proportion is the relationship between quantities. It is set up as an equation and represents the equality of two ratios. It usually is written:

$$\frac{3}{7} = \frac{9}{21} \quad \text{or} \quad 3:7::9:21 \ (3:7 = 9:21).$$

In a **proportion** the quotient of the first ratio equals the quotient of the second ratio.

$$\text{Quotient of} \overbrace{}^{\text{Ratio}} = \text{Quotient of} \overbrace{}^{\text{Ratio}}$$

Using ratios given above, we can verify that their quotients are equal:

$$\frac{3}{7} = \frac{9}{21} \text{ reduces to } \frac{3}{7} = \frac{3}{7}$$

The ratios are equal and if divided would yield the same quotient.

We can now use this information to solve for an unknown quantity. Suppose that in 3 packages there is enough sugar to fill 7 teaspoons. If we want to have enough sugar to fill 21 teaspoons, how many packages are required? We can set up the following equation:

$$\frac{3 \text{ pkg}}{7 \text{ t}} = \frac{x \text{ pkg}}{21 \text{ t}}$$

The first ratio is set up from a specified ratio (relationship) presented in a problem situation.

The second ratio will contain one unknown item x. The section of the ratio in which the unknown is placed is determined by the first ratio. If the package is on the top in the first ratio, it must be so in the second ratio—the items (labeling) positionwise *must* match on both sides of the equation.

To solve this problem, we "cross multiply" (i.e., multiply the numerator of the first fraction by the denominator of the second fraction and the denominator of the first fraction by the numerator of the second fraction):

$$\frac{3}{7} \diagdown\diagup \frac{x}{21}$$

$7x = 3 \times 21$

$7x = 63$

[It is a good habit to place the unknown quantity (x) on the left side of the equals sign.]

$$x = \frac{63}{7} = 9 \text{ pkg}$$

(To solve for x divide each side of the equation by the number next to the x.)

The answer obtained (9) can be checked for accuracy by putting it into the proportion where the x was:

$$\frac{3}{7}\times\frac{x}{21} \rightarrow \frac{3}{7} = \frac{9}{21}$$

We then cross multiply; if 9 is the correct answer, the products on each side of the equals sign will be equal:

$$\frac{3}{7} = \frac{9}{21}$$

$$3 \times 21 = 7 \times 9$$

$$63 = 63 \checkmark$$

Another way to verify that 9 is the correct answer is simply to divide the numerator and denominator of

$$\frac{9}{21} \text{ by 3, which confirms that } \frac{9}{21} = \frac{3}{7}.$$

The other acceptable way of writing a proportion for the problem we just discussed is

$$3 \text{ pkg}:7 \text{ t} :: x \text{ pkg}:21 \text{ t}$$

If this method is chosen, the cross multiplication is between the inner and outer positions, or "the product of the means equals the product of the extremes":

3 pkg:7 t :: x pkg:21 t   (Be sure positions of labels are the same—pkg:t::pkg:t.)

Means (inner positions)
Extremes (outer positions)

$7x = 3 \times 21$ (Keep the unknown quantity to the left side.)

$7x = 63$

$x = \dfrac{63}{7} = 9 \text{ pkg}$ (To solve for x, divide each side of the equation by the number next to the x.)

To prove or verify the answer, substitute in the answer and multiply; if correct, the product of means will equal the product of the extremes:

$$3 \text{ pkg}:7 \text{ t}::9 \text{ pkg}:21 \text{ t}$$

$$7 \times 9 = 3 \times 21$$
$$63 = 63 \checkmark$$

Practice Problems

Write proportions for the following:

156. There are 6 patients assigned to each nurse. How many nurses will be needed to take care of 96 patients?

157. There are 13 vitamin pills in 1 bottle. Each patient must receive 2 per day. There are 39 patients on the unit. How many bottles must you have available for the day?

158. If there are 60 mg in 1 pill and you must give 30 mg, how many pills will you give?

159. If 25 mg are in 5 cc, how many mg are in $\frac{1}{2}$ cc?

Solve the following:

160. $\dfrac{5}{9} = \dfrac{x}{90}$

161. $\dfrac{7}{8} = \dfrac{49}{x}$

162. $\dfrac{\frac{1}{4}}{1} = \dfrac{\frac{1}{8}}{x}$

163. $\dfrac{10}{1.8} = \dfrac{x}{0.54}$

164. $1:4::5:x$

165. $1:x::0.25:8$

166. $6:x = 10:16$

167. $\dfrac{1}{3}:x = \dfrac{3}{4}:\dfrac{9}{10}$

Answers for Chapter 3

PRACTICE PROBLEMS

1. $\dfrac{8}{11}$

2. $\dfrac{8}{13}$

3. $\dfrac{18}{19}$

4. $\dfrac{7}{38}$

5. $\dfrac{13}{14}$

6. $\dfrac{19}{45}$

7. $\dfrac{13}{21}$

8. $3\dfrac{7}{10}$

9. $3\dfrac{11}{15}$

10. $4\dfrac{10}{12}$ or $4\dfrac{5}{6}$

11. $\dfrac{3}{13}$

12. $\dfrac{7}{18}$

13. $\dfrac{3}{19}$

14. $\dfrac{7}{18}$

15. $\dfrac{6}{21}$ or $\dfrac{2}{7}$

16. $\dfrac{5}{21}$

17. $2\dfrac{4}{9}$

18. $4\dfrac{2}{13}$

19. $2\dfrac{3}{4}$

20. $1\dfrac{17}{21}$

21. $\dfrac{1}{2}$

22. $\dfrac{1}{2}$

23. $\dfrac{2}{3}$

24. $\dfrac{1}{3}$

25. $\dfrac{1}{4}$

26. $2\dfrac{5}{8}$

27. $2\dfrac{4}{7}$

28. $1\dfrac{1}{2}$

29. $1\dfrac{1}{4}$

30. $2\dfrac{1}{2}$

31. $\dfrac{17}{6}$

32. $\dfrac{53}{10}$

33. $\dfrac{56}{9}$

34. $\dfrac{37}{8}$

35. $\dfrac{14}{9}$

36. $\dfrac{3}{8}$

37. $\dfrac{1}{16}$

38. $\dfrac{7}{30}$

39. $\dfrac{2}{63}$

40. $\dfrac{1}{12}$

41. $\dfrac{2}{7}$

42. $\dfrac{1}{16}$

43. $\dfrac{4}{17}$

44. $\dfrac{1}{9}$

45. $\dfrac{8}{31}$

46. $4\frac{1}{2}$ 47. 2   48. $\frac{2}{3}$

49. $1\frac{1}{4}$ 50. $\frac{1}{3}$ 51. $1\frac{1}{8}$

52. 1   53. $1\frac{3}{7}$ 54. $\frac{13}{30}$

55. $1\frac{2}{7}$ 56. $2\frac{2}{3}$ 57. $\frac{2}{15}$

58. 4   59. $2\frac{3}{4}$ 60. $2\frac{5}{8}$

61. 64   62. 9   63. $\frac{1}{100}$

64. $\frac{1}{441}$ 65. 1   66. $\frac{1}{2}, \frac{1}{3}, \frac{1}{4}, \frac{1}{8}$

67. $\frac{2}{5}, \frac{3}{10}, \frac{6}{25}, \frac{1}{100}$ 68. $\frac{3}{8}, \frac{1}{4}, \frac{3}{32}, \frac{1}{16}$ 69. $\frac{1}{2}, \frac{7}{18}, \frac{1}{3}, \frac{1}{6}$

70. One hundred thousand and three tenths; $100,000\frac{3}{10}$

71. Fifteen thousand and twenty-seven hundredths; $15,000\frac{27}{100}$

72. Two thousand and one hundred forty-nine thousandths; $2,000\frac{149}{1000}$

73. Five hundred and five hundred thirty-four ten thousandths; $500\frac{534}{10,000}$

74. Seven and twenty-three thousandths; $7\frac{23}{1000}$

75. Three hundredths; $\frac{3}{100}$

76. Fifteen and fifteen hundred thousandths; $15\frac{15}{100,000}$

77. 5.00003, $5\frac{3}{100,000}$ 78. 0.0227, $\frac{227}{10,000}$

79. 15.05, $15\frac{5}{100} \rightarrow 15\frac{1}{20}$ 80. 6.6, $6\frac{6}{10} \rightarrow 6\frac{3}{5}$

81. 0.007, $\frac{7}{1000}$ 82. 9.0009, $9\frac{9}{10,000}$ 83. 0.123, $\frac{123}{1000}$

84. 100,000.7; one hundred thousand and seven tenths
85. 1.87; one and eighty-seven hundredths

86. 13.527; thirteen and five hundred twenty-seven thousandths
87. 0.0037; thirty-seven ten thousandths
88. 0.00127; one hundred twenty-seven hundred thousandths

89. 0.03	90. 0.2	91. 0.107
92. 0.5	93. 0.5	94. 5.1
95. 5.23	96. 927.0401	97. 19.9004
98. 35.751	99. 11.1556	100. 23.2681
101. 1.08	102. 5.06	103. 10.4
104. 3.156	105. 100.014	106. 5.112
107. 0.28	108. 0.3744	109. 4.9
110. 0.25	111. 0.0625	112. 3.02
113. 1.05	114. 1	115. 1
116. 2.02	117. 0.3333	118. 0.125
119. 0.0625	120. 0.06	121. 0.08

122. 0.75, 0.425, 0.275, 0.08, 0.0109
123. 1.0, 0.8, 0.45, 0.325, 0.052
124. 0.54, 0.054, 0.0054, 0.00054
125. 0.75, 0.66, 0.33, 0.25
126. 0.5, 0.25, 0.125, 0.05
127. 6.30. = 630
128. 35.35 = 0.3535
129. 3.75 = 37.5
130. .3.75 = 0.375
131. 15.957. = 15957
132. .015.957 = 0.015957
133. 33. = 0.33
134. 33.00. = 3300
135. $\dfrac{13}{100}$, 0.13
136. $\dfrac{30}{100}$ = $\dfrac{3}{10}$, 0.3
137. $\dfrac{25}{100}$ = $\dfrac{1}{4}$, 0.25
138. $\dfrac{1}{100}$, 0.01
139. $\dfrac{15}{100}$ = $\dfrac{3}{20}$, 0.15

140. 70

141. 7.2

142. 25

143. 9

144. 12.5

145. 5

146. 10

147. 75

148. 80

149. 90

150. 60

151. 9

152. $\dfrac{7}{13}$, 7:13

153. $\dfrac{1}{6}$, 1:6

154. $\dfrac{5}{7}$, 5:7

155. $\dfrac{4}{9}$, 4:9

156. 6 pt:1 N::96 pt:x N   or $\dfrac{6 \text{ pt}}{1 \text{ N}} = \dfrac{96 \text{ pt}}{x \text{ N}}$

157. 13 pills:1 bottle:: 78 pills:x bottles   or $\dfrac{13 \text{ pills}}{1 \text{ bottle}} = \dfrac{78 \text{ pills}}{x \text{ bottles}}$

158. 60 mg:1 pill::30 mg:x pill   or $\dfrac{60 \text{ mg}}{1 \text{ pill}} = \dfrac{30 \text{ mg}}{x \text{ pill}}$

159. 25 mg:5 cc::x mg:$\dfrac{1}{2}$ cc   or $\dfrac{25 \text{ mg}}{5 \text{ cc}} = \dfrac{x \text{ mg}}{\dfrac{1}{2} \text{ cc}}$

160. 50

161. 56

162. $\dfrac{1}{2}$

163. 3

164. 20

165. 32

166. 9.6

167. $\dfrac{2}{5}$

4 | *Metric Measures*

Terminal Performance Objectives

1. Given a dosage order written in a basic unit of the metric system, the reader is able to compute the number of tablets or cubic centimeters (or milliliters) of medication to be administered.

2. Given a dosage order written in a basic unit of the metric system, the reader is able to convert it into the subunits of that system and compute the number of tablets or cubic centimeters (or milliliters) of medication to be administered.

3. Given a dosage order written in the subunits of the metric system, the reader is able to convert it into a basic unit of that system and compute the number of tablets or cubic centimeters (or milliliters) of medication to be administered.

4. Given a dosage order in a subunit of the metric system, the reader is able to convert it into other subunits of the system and compute the number of cubic centimeters (or milliliters) or tablets to be administered.

5. Given a selection of tablets or liquid preparations of various strengths in the metric system, the reader is able to select the most appropriate strength and compute the number of tablets or cubic centimeters (or milliliters) to be administered.

6. Given an available liquid preparation's strength, the reader is able to compute the amount of active ingredient in the individual vehicle unit.

7. Given what the drug literature states is the recommended dosage per kilogram of body weight and the patient's weight in kilograms, the reader is able to calculate the amount of medication the patient should receive.

8. Given the recommended dosage and the patient's weight, the reader is able to determine if a prescribed dose lies within the stipulated safety range.

9. Given a prescribed dose to administer, the reader is able to indicate on a diagram of either a medicine cup or a syringe the amount of liquid volume to give.

10. Given an injectable medication in powdered form, the reader is mathematically able to prepare it into a solution form, label its strength per cubic centimeter (or milliliter), and calculate the amount of fluid to be withdrawn for a prescribed dose.

INTERMEDIATE PERFORMANCE OBJECTIVES

After studying the content in this chapter pertaining to the calculation of drug dosages, the reader is able to do the following:

1. List the basic unit and the subunits of the liquid measures of the metric system.

2. List the basic unit and subunits of the measures of weight of the metric system.

3. Write the meaning of a given abbreviation in the metric system.

4. Write the abbreviation for the basic unit and the subunits of the metric system.

5. Write the equivalents of a given unit or subunit of the metric system.

6. Define the rule to convert liters to milliliters (or cubic centimeters).

7. Convert liters to milliliters (or cubic centimeters)

8. Define the rule to convert milliliters (or cubic centimeters) to liters.

9. Convert milliliters (or cubic centimeters) to liters.

10. Add liters and milliliters (or cubic centimeters).

11. Define the rule to convert grams to milligrams.

12. Convert grams to milligrams.

13. Define the rule to convert milligrams to grams.

14. Convert milligrams to grams.

15. Define the rule to convert milligrams to micrograms.

16. Convert milligrams to micrograms.

17. Define the rule to convert micrograms to milligrams.

18. Convert micrograms to milligrams.

19. Use the proportion method to calculate the number of tablets or cubic centimeters (or milliliters) for a prescribed dose.

20. Use the formula method to calculate the number of tablets or cubic centimeters (or milliliters) for a prescribed dose.

21. Identify the active ingredient as opposed to the vehicle in a given statement on dosages.

22. Read the calibration lines on four commonly used syringes (the 2 to 3 cc, 5 cc, 10 cc, and the tuberculin syringe).

23. State the name of the syringe that provides for fine measurement of fluid volume dosages of tenths of a cubic centimeter (or milliliter).

24. State the average amount of fluid volume that is administered via the intramuscular and subcutaneous routes.

25. State the fact that the more diluted a prescribed medication dose is, the less irritating it is and the more rapidly it will be absorbed, leading to a quicker onset of action.

26. State three solutions that the medication literature may cite as the appropriate diluents to be utilized for injectable medications.

27. List the sequence of steps that would be followed in preparing a solution from a powdered form, when the medication is accompanied by dilution instruction information.

28. Select, from a given dilution table, the appropriate dilution equivalent to be used.

29. Label a prepared solution, including the dilution strength, the date and time of preparation, the date and time of expiration, and the initials of the preparer.

30. Calculate the amount of fluid volume to be withdrawn from the above prepared solutions for a prescribed dose.

▶ After reading these objectives, if you feel confident about your knowledge in this area, take the pretest. If you know that you are not able to perform these behaviors, begin the metric system by reading and memorizing the data in the Introduction and the General Information section.

Pretest

TPO   IPO

1,2

1. List the basic units and subunits of the metric system for both liquid measures and measures of weight used in dosage calculations.

3,4

2. Write the meaning or give the abbreviation for the following:
   (a) _____ liter
   (b) _____ cubic centimeter
   (c) mL _____

5

3. Equivalents:

(a) 1 cc	= _____ mL		(b) 1 L	= _____ cc
(c) 1 L	= _____ mL		(d) 1000 cc	= _____ L
(e) 1000 mL	= _____ L		(f) 1 mL	= _____ cc

6,8

4. (a) State the rule to convert liters to milliliters.
   (b) State the rule to convert milliliters to liters.

7,9

5. Convert:

(a) 4.0 l	= _____ mL	(b) 400 mL	= _____ L
(c) 6.75 l	= _____ cc	(d) 3050 cc	= _____ L
(e) 520 cc	= _____ L	(f) 1.7 L	= _____ cc
(g) 3000 mL	= _____ L	(h) 2.05 L	= _____ mL

10

6. (a) 5 L + 45 cc + 175 mL + 3.6 L + 0.3 L = _____ cc
   (b) 4 L + 30 cc + 200 mL + 4.5 L + 0.4 L = _____ L

11,13
15,17

7. (a) State the rule to convert grams to milligrams.
   (b) State the rule to convert milligrams to grams.
   (c) State the rule to convert milligrams to micrograms.
   (d) State the rule to convert micrograms to milligrams.

12,14

8. Convert:

(a) 1 g	= _____ mg	(b) 500 mg	= _____ g
(c) 1.25 g	= _____ mg	(d) 650 mg	= _____ g
(e) 1 mg	= _____ g	(f) 1.7 g	= _____ mg
(g) 740 mg	= _____ g	(h) 0.3 g	= _____ mg

TPO	IPO
	16,18

9. Convert:
   (a) 1 mg   = _____ mcg   (b) 0.275 mg = _____ mcg
   (c) 450 mcg   = _____ mg   (d) 0.03 mg   = _____ mcg
   (e) 300 mcg   = _____ mg   (f) 0.8 mg   = _____ mcg
   (g) 0.375 mg   = _____ mcg   (h) 4000 mcg = _____ mg

	21

10. In each description in the following list identify the notation that refers to the active ingredient (the medication component) and those that refer to the vehicle (the preparation form) that contains it:
    (a) 10 mcg per tablet   (b) 500 mg per 5 cc
    (c) 500 cc contains 60 g   (d) 1 capsule is 250 mcg
    (e) 1 g/cc

1	19

11. A medicine is available as 0.5 g/cc and you must administer 0.625 g. You will give _____ cc. (To calculate, use the proportion method.)

1	19

12. A medicine is available as 0.005 g per tablet and you must administer 0.01 g. You will give _____ tablet(s). (Use the proportion method.)

2	20

13. A medication is available as 700 mg/cc and you must administer 0.35 g. You will give _____ cc. (To calculate, use the formula method.)

1	20

14. A medicine is available as 0.5 g per tablet and you must administer 0.25 g. You will give _____ tablet(s). (Use the formula method.)

3	19 or 20

15. A drug is available as 0.5 g per 2 cc and you must give 125 mg. You will give _____ cc.

2	19 or 20

16. A drug is available as 45 mg per tablet and you must administer 0.09 g. You will give _____ tablet(s).

3	19 or 20

17. A medicine comes 2 g per 8 cc and you must administer 125 mg. You will give _____ cc.

3	19 or 20

18. A drug is diluted as 1.5 g/L and you must administer 375 mg. How much fluid volume in cubic centimeters will this person receive?

6	19

19. A drug is mixed as 2 g per 0.5 L. How many milligrams are there in 1 cc?

	7,9,10

20. A woman's fluid intake consisted of soup (0.12 L), coffee (200 cc), juice (90 mL), and ice cream (0.15 L). Her total fluid intake for that meal was _____ L.

TPO	IPO	
2	19 or 20	21. You must administer 0.75 g. The medicine is available as 375 mg per tablet. You will give _____ tablet(s).
4	19 or 20	22. A doctor's order reads: administer 0.125 mg by mouth. The liquid preparation available is 25 mcg per 5 cc. You will give _____ cc.
4	19 or 20	23. The doctor orders 1250 mcg in a liquid preparation to be taken by mouth. The solution is available as 0.25 mg per 5 cc. You will administer _____ cc.
5	19 or 20	24. You must administer 0.5 mg. You find the following tablets available: 2.5 mg, 0.25 mg, 0.125 mg, 0.01 mg, and 1.0 mg. You should administer _____ of the _____ tablet(s).
5	19 or 20	25. You must administer 0.625 g. You find the following oral solutions available: 0.125 mg per 5 cc, 6.25 mg per 5 cc, 62.5 mg per 5 cc, 125 mg per 5 cc, and 25 mg per 5 cc. You should administer _____ .
7		26. Drug literature states that the recommended dose is 6 mg/kg of body weight. The patient weighs 66 kg. This person should receive ____ mg?
7	15,16	27. Drug data states that the recommended dose is 30 mcg/kg of body weight. The patient weighs 75 kg. The patient must receive _____ mg.
8		28. A recommended drug dose is 4 mg/kg of body weight in four equally divided doses. The patient weighs 100 kg. The prescribed order reads for you to administer 100 mg q.i.d. Is this order appropriate?
8		29. A recommended dose is 150 mg/kg/day. The patient weighs 75 kg and is receiving 3.75 g q8h. Is this drug order appropriate?
9	11,19, or 20	30. A drug is available as 500 mg per 5 cc and you must administer 1 g. Draw an arrow to indicate the amount of fluid volume you would pour into this cup to administer this dosage.

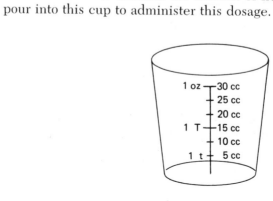

TPO   IPO
9   22,23

31. A drug is available as 10 mg/cc and you must administer 7 mg. Draw the type of syringe you would use and place an arrow to indicate the amount of fluid volume you would prepare in the syringe to administer this dose.

10   24–30

32. Prescribed dose: 100 mg IM. In reference to the directions below:
    (a) What diluent should be used?
    (b) What solution strength would you select?
    (c) How much fluid volume would you administer intramuscularly?
    (d) What would you write on the bottle label after you have prepared this?

DIRECTIONS

1. Use sterile normal saline for injection as the diluent.
2. Follow the dilution table below.
3. Use within 24 hours after being prepared into a solution form.

Active Ingredient in Container	Recommended Amount of Diluent to Add	Total Fluid Volume	Concentration
(a) 1 g	1.8 cc	2 cc	500 mg/cc
(b) 2 g	3.6 cc	4 cc	500 mg/cc
(c) 500 mg	8.4 cc	10 cc	50 mg/cc
(d) 250 mg	0.9 cc	1 cc	250 mg/cc
(e) 50 mg	0.8 cc	1 cc	50 mg/cc

▶ Compare your answers with those listed at the end of this chapter. If you have mastered this test, then you may bypass this chapter and begin the next chapter. If you have not mastered this test, proceed to memorize the data that follows.

INTRODUCTION

In the calculation of drug dosages, the major system of measurement is the metric system. Therefore, this is the system that is emphasized in this text. In the past, the apothecary system was frequently used for drug measurement. For many years, however, it has decreased in usage because it is not as precise a system of measurement as the metric system. If you need to learn the apothecary system, Part III of this text provides ample practice to make you quite proficient with this system as well as to be able to use it interchangeably with the metric system and household measures.

You are probably familiar with aspects of the metric system from your previous studies. Because only a portion of the metric system is employed in the calculation of drug dosages, only the pertinent parts of this system are included in this text. This will help you focus on the relevant aspects and facilitate in-depth learning.

In the calculation of drug dosages you will be concerned with only the smaller units of measurement of the metric system, for often a very small amount of drug produces an extremely potent effect; large amounts are rarely utilized. You will also frequently use the units of weight and volume in your calculations; therefore, these units are emphasized. Linear measure is not frequently encountered, except perhaps when graphs are employed for children's dosages. Such relevant data are discussed later in the text.

Lastly, the metric system uses decimals for fractional amounts; therefore, be sure you are able to work with skill with decimals. The following text organizes the data you need to know about the metric system.

GENERAL INFORMATION

In the calculation of drug dosages, it is helpful if you think of every medication in terms of two aspects: (1) the active ingredient (the substance that makes the drug work), and (2) the vehicle (the preparation form in which the medication is available), as is shown in the following figure:

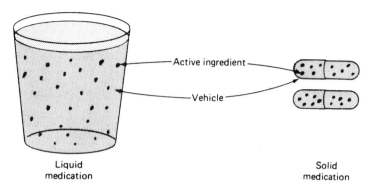

Medication comes in both liquid and solid form.

Generally not all parts of a liquid or solid preparation are actually medicine. The active ingredient of a medication is usually measured in terms of a weight or concentration factor, as is shown in the figure below.

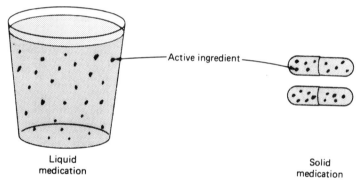

In the metric system the active ingredient is measured in grams (g), milligrams (mg), or micrograms (mcg).

In the metric system, the weight factors used are the gram (g), milligram (mg), and microgram (mcg). This also is how a drug is usually ordered, for example, administer 50 mg.

Vehicles (preparation forms) can be either liquid or solid in form, as is shown in the following figure. Typical dry or solid forms of vehicles are tablets, capsules, or spansules. The units for liquid measurement in the metric system are the liter (L) and the milliliter (mL) or cubic centimeter (cc). Note that 1 mL = 1 cc—milliliters and cubic centimeters are therefore used interchangeably throughout this text.

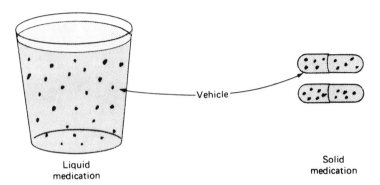

Liquid
medication

Solid
medication

Vehicle

In all systems the solid vehicle is in such forms as spansules, capsules, or
tablets. In the metric system the liquid vehicle is measured in liters (L) and
milliliters (mL) or cubic centimeters (cc).

The important aspect to remember in all of this is that every medication be it liquid or solid in form is actually not all medicine. Only a
portion of it is. The other portion is an inactive ingredient. In calculating
accurate drug dosages, one must ensure that the proper amount of a
preparation is administered in order to assure the administration of an
accurate amount of medicine (active ingredient).

READING OF A DRUG LABEL

Every medication that you use will bear a label stating the amount of
active ingredient and the specified amount of vehicle. Here are two examples. Note that they are both the same drug but there is a different
amount of medication per milliliter.

Active Ingredient	Specified Amount/Vehicle
(a) 5 mg	mL
(b) 8 mg	mL

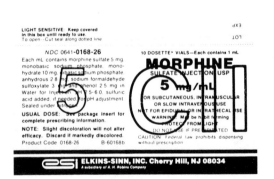

(a)

(b)

GUIDE TO BE USED DURING DRUG PREPARATION

When you have a choice among tablet preparations of various strengths for a given dose, avoid the splitting of tablets, if possible, and choose the least number of them to administer the prescribed dose. However, if you must split a tablet, remember to do this only with scored preparations.

When administering liquid preparations, the following is a useful guide to the typical prescribed amounts: oral—5 to 30 cc; intramuscular injection—up to 3 cc (1 to 2 cc most common); and subcutaneous injections—1 cc or less.

▶   When you are confident of this material, complete Activity Sheet 1.

Activity Sheet 1

1. What is the major system of measurement used in the calculation of drug dosages?

2. Will you use the smaller or larger units of metric measurement in calculating drug dosages?

3. Which two of the following will you use most frequently in calculating drug dosages: weight, volume, or linear measurement?

4. Which system of measurement is more accurate—the apothecary or the metric?

5. Which system of measurement is increasing in use in the United States?

6. Does the metric system utilize fractions or decimals?

7. What is an active ingredient?

8. What is a vehicle?

9. What three weight factors in the metric system are utilized to measure the active ingredient of a medicine?

10. Name the typical units in which liquid vehicles are measured in the metric system.

11. Name some typical units for dry or solid vehicles.

12. The following are examples of medication labels. For each, state the amount of active ingredient and the vehicle/preparation form.

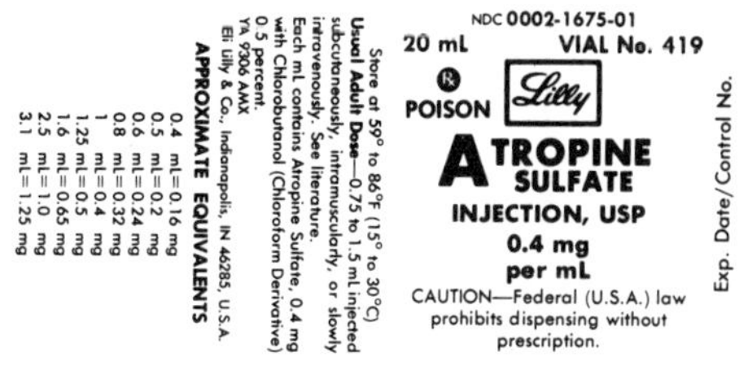

(a)

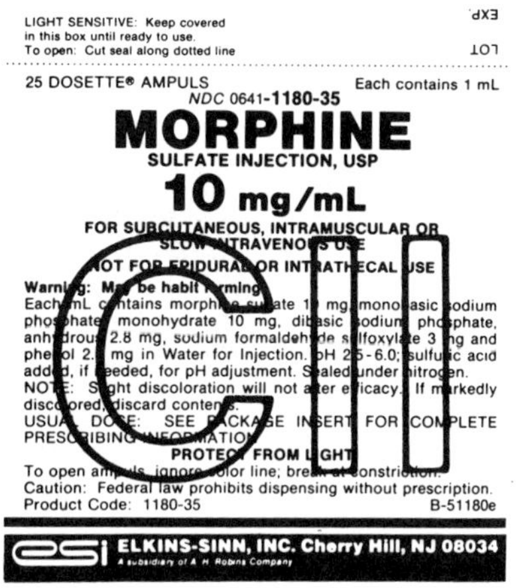

(b)

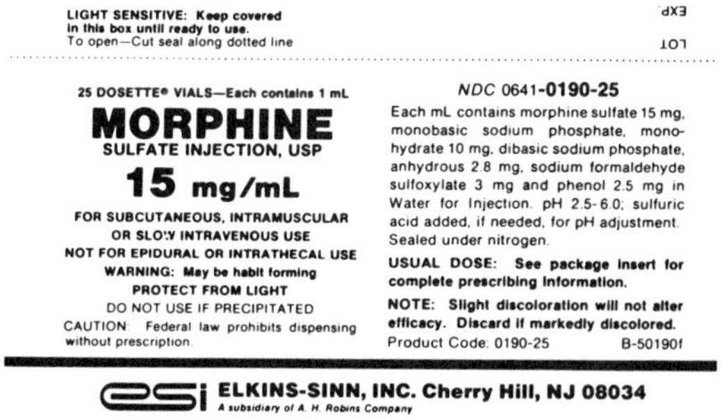

(c)

13. When you have the choice of tablet preparations of various strengths for a specified dosage, what factors should you consider?

14. List the usual amount of liquid ordered to be administered by the following routes: (a) oral, (b) intramuscular, and (c) subcutaneous.

▶ Compare your answers with the answer sheet at the end of this chapter. If you have mastered Activity Sheet 1 (you have answered with 100% accuracy), proceed to read and memorize the data in the next section. If you did not master this activity sheet, review the previous text and redo the incorrect problems. Then proceed to the next section.

METRIC SYSTEM: CONVERTING LIQUID MEASURES

- Basic unit: Liter
- Subunit: Milliliter or cubic centimeter

Abbreviations: *Equivalents:*
Liter = L, l, ℓ   1 L ↔ 1000 mL
Milliliter = mL, ml, mℓ   1 cc ↔   1 mL
Cubic centimeters = cc

- In the metric system abbreviations are now frequently being written without the period following the abbreviation. Be aware that abbreviations are written in both capital and small letters. The capital letter L is used throughout this book because lowercase l can be confused with the number one (1). You will use the data on converting metric measures not only in calculating drug dosages but also in the administration of intravenous solutions and in calculating a person's intake and output of fluid.

Liters ▶ Milliliters

- To convert liters to milliliters multiply by 1000.
- Move decimal point 3 places to the right .
- *Note:* 1 cc = 1 mL

Examples:

3 L = 3.000. or 3,000 mL

6.5 L = 6.500. or 6,500 mL

4.9 L = 4.900. or 4,900 mL

4.75 L = 4.750. or 4,750 mL

Milliliters ▶ Liters

- To convert milliliters to liters divide by 1000.
- Move decimal point 3 places to the left.
- *Note:* 1 cc = 1 mL

Examples:

6000 mL = 6.000. or 6   L

500 mL = 0.500. or 0.5   L

7500 mL = 7.500. or 7.5 L

450 mL = .450. or 0.45 L

▶ When you feel confident about the data on this page, proceed on and complete Activity Sheet 2.

Activity Sheet 2

1. List the basic unit(s) of metric liquid measure.

2. List the subunit(s) of metric liquid measure.

3. Abbreviate or write the meaning for the following:
   (a) milliliter = _____
   (b) _____ = cc
   (c) liter = _____

4. (a) One liter equals how many milliliters?
   (b) One thousand cubic centimeters equal how many liters?

5. State the rule to convert liters to milliliters and/or cubic centimeters.

6. Convert:
   (a) 2 L = 2._____ mL   (b) 0.3 L = 0.3 _____ cc
   (c) 0.12 L = 0.12_____ mL   (d) 3.62 L = 3.62_____ mL
   (e) 1.30 L = 1.30 _____ cc   (f) 2.4 L = _____ cc
   (g) 0.009 L = _____ mL   (h) 5 L = _____ cc
   (i) 0.15 L = _____ mL   (j) 0.5 L = _____ cc

7. State the rule to convert milliliters or cubic centimeters to liters.

8. Convert:
   (a) 325 cc = 325. L   (b) 50 mL = 50. L
   (c) 2500 cc = 2500. L   (d) 175 mL = 175. L
   (e) 3020 cc = 3020. L   (f) 250 cc = _____ L
   (g) 3600 mL = _____ L   (h) 4570 cc = _____ L
   (i) 75 mL = _____ L   (j) 750 cc = _____ L

9. Mr. S. is to receive 2500 cc of fluids. How many liters is this?

10. Mr. S. drank 400 cc of fluid for breakfast, 500 cc for lunch, 450 cc for supper, and 250 cc at bedtime as a snack.
    (a) How many milliliters is this?
    (b) How many liters is this?

11. If a patient is to receive 1250 cc of fluid by mouth and 1500 cc through other routes, how much does this total in liters for that day?

12. You must assure that a patient receives 3.5 L in 24 hours. How many milliliters is this?

13. A patient receives 0.25 L for breakfast, 0.3 L for lunch, 0.5 L for supper, 0.75 L with pills, and 0.125 L for a bedtime snack. How many cubic centimeters did this person drink?

14. Mr. M's fluid intake yesterday was as follows: intravenously, 1.5 L; and orally, 300 cc for breakfast, 0.25 L for lunch, 275 cc for supper, and 175 mL with pills. What is the patient's total intake in liters?

15. A patient's fluid output is 1.5 L of urine and 0.75 L through other means (tubes, liquid feces, and so on). How many cubic centimeters is this?

▶   Compare your answers with the answer sheet at the end of this chapter. If you have answered the questions in Activity Sheet 2 with 100% accuracy proceed to read and memorize the data in the next section. If you did not master this activity sheet, review the previous text and redo the incorrect problems. Then proceed to the next section.

METRIC SYSTEM: CONVERTING MEASURES OF WEIGHT—SECTION A

- Basic unit: Gram
- Subunits: Milligram, microgram

Abbreviations:[a]	Equivalents:
Gram = g, gm, G, Gm	1 g ↔ 1000 mg
Milligram = mg, mgm	1 mg ↔ 1000 mcg
Microgram = mcg, μg, mcgm	

[a] *Note:* In the metric system these abbreviations are frequently written using small letters and without a period following the abbreviation.

Grams ▶ Milligrams

- To convert grams to milligrams multiply by 1000
- Move the decimal point 3 places to the right

Examples:

2.0 g = 2.000. = 2000 mg

0.5 g = 0.500. = 500 mg

1.25 g = 1.250. = 1250 mg

0.03 g = 0.030. = 30 mg

Milligrams ▶ Grams

- To convert milligrams to grams divide by 1000
- Move the decimal point 3 places to the left

Examples:

4000 mg = 4.000. = 4   g

50 mg = 0.050. = 0.05 g

250 mg = 0.250. = 0.25 g

600 mg = 0.600. = 0.6 g

METRIC SYSTEM: CONVERTING MEASURES OF WEIGHT—SECTION B

- Amounts less than 1.0 mg are usually written as a decimal of the unit, milligrams rather than in micrograms.
- If, however, you have to convert between these two measures (mg and mcg), follow the guide below.

Equivalents: 1 mg ↔ 1000 mcg

Milligrams ▶ Micrograms

- To convert milligrams to micrograms multiply by 1000.
- Move the decimal point 3 places to the right.
- *Note:* mcg = µg.

Examples:

0.1	mg =	0.100.	=	100 mcg
0.5	mg =	0.500.	=	500 µg
0.01	mg =	0.010.	=	10 µg
0.065	mg =	0.065.	=	65 mcg
0.75	mg =	0.750.	=	750 µg

Micrograms ▶ Milligrams

- To convert micrograms to milligrams divide by 1000.
- Move the decimal point 3 places to the left.
- *Note:* mcg = µg.

Examples:

350 µg	=	0.350.	=	0.35 mg
400 mcg	=	0.400.	=	0.4 mg
25 µg	=	0.025.	=	0.025 mg
500 mcg	=	0.500.	=	0.5 mg
5 µg	=	0.005.	=	0.005 mg

▶ When you feel confident about the contents of sections A and B, complete Activity Sheet 3.

Activity Sheet 3

1. List the basic unit(s) of the metric system of weight used in dosage calculations.

2. List the subunit(s) of the metric system of weight used in dosage calculations.

3. Write the abbreviation(s) or the term for the following (where the term is given, write all the abbreviations that might be used for it):
   - (a) g   = _____
   - (b) mcg   = _____
   - (c) mg   = _____
   - (d) microgram = _____
   - (e) gram   = _____
   - (f) milligram = _____

4. Write the equivalent:
   - (a) 1 g   = _____ mg
   - (b) 1 mg   = _____ mcg
   - (c) 1000 mcg = _____ mg
   - (d) 1000 mg   = _____ g

5. What is the rule to convert grams to milligrams?

6. What is the rule to convert milligrams to grams?

7. Convert the following:
   - (a) 100 mg   = _____ g
   - (b) 10 mg   = _____ g
   - (c) 1500 mg = _____ g
   - (d) 0.006 g   = _____ mg
   - (e) 0.065 g   = _____ mg
   - (f) 0.05 g   = _____ mg
   - (g) 30 mg   = _____ g
   - (h) 850 mg   = _____ g
   - (i) 4 mg   = _____ g
   - (j) 250 mg   = _____ g
   - (k) 750 mg   = _____ g
   - (l) 1.7 g   = _____ mg
   - (m) 3.62 g   = _____ mg
   - (n) 1000 mg   = _____ g

8. State the rule to convert milligrams to micrograms.

9. State the rule to convert micrograms to milligrams.

10. Convert the following:
    (a) 150 mcg = _____ mg   (b) 800 mcg = _____ mg
    (c) 0.9 mg   = _____ mcg   (d) 0.125 mg = _____ mcg
    (e) 5000 mcg = _____ mg   (f) 0.375 mg = _____ mcg
    (g) 250 mcg = _____ mg   (h) 0.05 mg = _____ mcg
    (i) 405 mcg = _____ mg   (j) 1000 mcg = _____ mg

► Compare your answers with those at the end of this chapter. If you have answered the questions in Activity Sheet 3 with 100% accuracy, proceed to read and memorize the data in the next section. If you have not mastered this activity sheet, review the previous text in this chapter and redo the questions you answered incorrectly. Then go on to read the next section.

PROBLEM SOLVING

You will find that there are many ways to solve problems of drug dosages. We look here at two of the most common and easiest methods. Some people prefer a formula. Some prefer the ratio–proportion method, for they have used it for years and therefore will not have to memorize a formula. The method of problem solving you choose is up to you. Whichever method you employ, your answers should be the same as the answers given in this text. You will find, however, that with many problems you will have to use the ratio–proportion method even though you prefer the formula method. Regardless of the problem-solving method you use, you should always perform the problem-solving steps described below— steps 1 and 2—in order to organize the data that are known to you.

Example

A medication is available and labeled 0.09 g/cc, and you must administer 45 mg. How much will you administer?

To Solve
1. *Isolate the known facts:*

Dose on hand: 0.09 g/cc

Desired dose: 45 mg/x cc

When you write out these quantities, always keep the active ingredient to one side and the vehicle to the other.
2. *Check the quantities:* They must be at the same value level within the same system.

Active ingredients: In this example the quantities are in the same system but at different levels—45 mg is at one level and 0.09 g is at another. In this example we can easily change 0.09 g to 90 mg, and we now say that we have available 90 mg/cc.

Vehicles: In inspecting the vehicles we see that they are in the same system and at the same level, both in cubic centimeters.

Review of the Ratio–Proportion Method
1. Proportion is a relationship between quantities:

$$\text{Quotient of } \frac{\text{first}}{\text{second}} = \text{Quotient of } \frac{\text{third}}{\text{fourth}}$$

2. Proportion is the equality of two ratios:

$$A:B::C:D \text{ or } A:B = C:D$$

Example

1. Relationship between quantities:

$$\frac{5}{15} = \frac{8}{24}$$

$$\frac{1}{3} = \frac{1}{3}$$

The quotients on either side of the equals sign are the same.

2. Equality of two ratios:

$$A:B = C:D$$

$$1:4 = 4:16$$

Each side of the equals sign has the same relationship. The second sections (B and D) are four times larger than the first sections (A and C).

Both of the above examples are mathematically valid; therefore one can solve a problem for an unknown quantity by using either of these methods.

Application of the Ratio–Proportion Method

Application of the ratio–proportion method to dosage problems should establish a relationship between the active ingredient and the vehicle of the dose on hand and the desired dose:

$$\frac{\text{Active ingredient in dose on hand}}{\text{Vehicle of dose on hand}} = \frac{\text{Active ingredient in desired dose}}{\text{Vehicle of desired dose}}$$

or

Active ingredient in dose on hand	:	Vehicle of dose on hand	::	Active ingredient in desired dose	:	Vehicle of desired dose

The relationship to the left of the equals sign, and the units in which the equation is stated are generally taken from the label of the medication available. Remember that a vehicle can be either liquid or solid in form.

Example

Dose on hand: 90 mg/cc

Desired dose: 45 mg

Using the information given above, calculate the number of cubic centimeters needed for the desired dose with (1) a relationship between quantities, and (2) the equality of two ratios.

First Method: Relationship Between Quantities

$$\frac{90 \text{ mg}}{1 \text{ cc}} = \frac{45 \text{ mg}}{x \text{ cc}}$$

As we have done here, always label the initial setup so that you can readily identify the units in which the answer will be expressed. Also keep relationships of both sets of quantities in the same order; here we have mg:cc, mg:cc.
Cross-multiply:

$$\frac{90}{1} \diagup\!\!\!\!\diagdown \frac{45}{x}$$

$$90x = 45$$

Solve for x by dividing each side of the equation by the number that is next to the x:

$$x = \frac{45}{90} = \frac{1}{2} \text{ cc} \quad \text{or} \quad 0.5 \text{ cc}$$

To prove that the answer is accurate, substitute the answer for x and cross-multiply:

$$\frac{90}{1} = \frac{45}{x}$$

$$\frac{90}{1} \diagup\!\!\!\!\diagdown \frac{45}{\frac{1}{2}}$$

$$90 \times \frac{1}{2} = 45 \times 1$$

$$45 = 45 \ \checkmark$$

The product on one side of the equals sign is equal to the product on the other side, proving the answer.

Second Method: Equality of Ratios

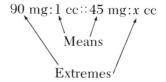

$$90 \text{ mg} : 1 \text{ cc} :: 45 \text{ mg} : x \text{ cc}$$

Means

Extremes

The product of the means equals the product of the extremes:

$$90x = 45$$

Solve for x by dividing each side of the equation by the number that is next to the x:

$$x = \frac{45}{90} = \frac{1}{2} \text{ cc} \quad \text{or} \quad 0.5 \text{ cc}$$

To prove that the answer is accurate, substitute the answer for x and the product of the means should equal the product of the extremes:

$$90:1 = 45:x$$

$$90:1 = 45:\frac{1}{2}$$

Means

Extremes

$$90 \times \frac{1}{2} = 45 \times 1$$

$$45 = 45 \checkmark$$

The product on one side of the equals sign is equal to the product on the other side, proving the answer.

Formula Method

Another means of solving this problem is the *formula method*:

Desired dose: 45 mg/x cc

Dose on hand: 90 mg/cc

Amount to administer

$$= \frac{\text{Desired dose}}{\text{Dose on hand}} \times \text{amount of vehicle per dose on hand}$$

$$= \frac{45 \text{ mg}}{90 \text{ mg}} \times 1 \text{ cc} = \frac{1}{2} \text{ cc or } 0.5 \text{ cc}$$

In deciding the label for the answer, look to the terms of the vehicle. Here it is given in cubic centimeters.

Summary

One can readily see that we actually used three different methods to solve this one dosage problem, and all three answers came out the same. In working through the subsequent problems you need not do them all three ways; simply choose the method that you find easiest.

▶ When you feel confident of the data in this section, solve the problems on Activity Sheet 4A.

Activity Sheet 4A

1. An oral liquid medication is available as 0.25 mg per 10 cc, and you must give a 0.125-mg dose. You will therefore give _____ cc.

2. An oral liquid medication is available as 35 mcg per 5 cc, and you must give 0.14 mg. You will administer _____ cc.

3. A drug is available as shown on the following morphine label, and you must administer 10 mg. How many cc (mL) will you give?

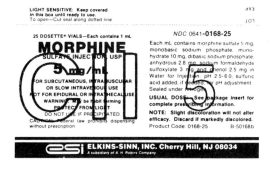

4. A drug comes 50 mg/cc, and you must administer 75 mg. You will give how many cc?

5. A drug comes 0.5 mg in 2 cc and you must give 0.125 mg. You will give how many cc?

6. A drug comes 0.5 g in 1 cc, and you must administer 1.25 g. How many cc will you give?

7. A medication is available as 0.25 g/cc, and you must administer 0.5 g. How many cc will you give?

8. A drug comes 250 mg/cc, and you must give 2.25 g. You must have how many cc?

73

9. A medication comes 0.5 g/cc, and you must give 750 mg. You will give how many mL?

10. You must give 0.75 mg of a drug, and the strength available is 1000 mcg/cc. How much fluid volume will you give?

11. If a drug comes 500 mcg/cc and you have to give 1.25 mg, you will give how much fluid volume?

12. If a medication comes 0.5 mg/cc and you must administer 0.625 mg, how much fluid volume will you give?

13. A medication comes as 0.2 mg per 2 cc, and you must administer 50 mcg. How much fluid volume will you give?

14. A medicine is available as 375 mcg per 2 cc, and you must administer 0.75 mg. How much fluid volume will you give?

15. You must give 0.375 mg, and it is available as 0.25 mg/cc. You will give _____ cc.

16. You must administer 0.125 g, and the medicine is available as 1500 mg in 12 cc. You will give _____ cc.

17. A medication is available as 10 mg/mL.

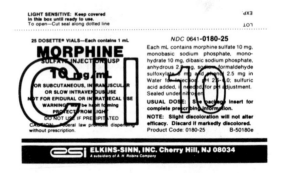

If you had to give 8 mg, you would give _____ mL. If you had to give 6 mg, you would give _____ mL.

18. You must prepare 2 doses of the following medication:

NDC 0002-1675-01
20 mL   VIAL No. 419

℞
POISON

ATROPINE
  SULFATE
INJECTION, USP

0.4 mg
per mL

Multiple Dose

CAUTION—Federal (U.S.A.)
law prohibits dispensing
without prescription.

Usual Adult Dose—0.75 to
1.5 mL injected subcuta-
neously, intramuscularly,
or slowly intravenously.

See accompanying
literature.

Store at Controlled Room
Temperature 59° to 86°F
(15° to 30°C)

Each mL contains Atropine
Sulfate, 0.4 mg with Chloro-
butanol (Chloroform Deriva-
tive) 0.5 percent as a pre-
servative, added at the time
of manufacture.

ELI LILLY AND COMPANY
Indianapolis, IN 46285, U.S.A.

(a) For a 0.28-mg dose, you will prepare _____ mL.
(b) For a 0.5-mg dose, you will prepare _____ mL.

▶   Do the problems on Activity Sheet 4B.

Activity Sheet 4B

In the following problems assume that the tablets are scored so that they can be divided, if necessary. (As you remember, only scored tablets should be divided.)

1. Tablets are available in 250 mg form:
   (a) To give 1000 mg, give _____ tablet(s).
   (b) To give 500 mg, give _____ tablet(s).

2. You must administer 250 mg of a medication, and the tablets are 0.5 g. How many will you give?

3. A drug comes 0.25 mg per tablet, and you must administer 0.125 mg. You will give _____ tablet(s).

4. You must administer 750 mg of a medication, which is available as 0.25 g per capsule. You will give _____ capsule(s).

5. A preparation comes as 0.25 mg per tablet, and you must give 0.5 mg. You will give _____ tablet(s).

6. You must give 1.5 g of a drug, and it is available as 750 mg per capsule. How many capsules will you give?

7. Tablets are available as 0.5 g, and you must administer 1000 mg. You will give _____ tablet(s).

8. Tablets come as 0.1 mg and you must administer 0.05 mg. You will give _____ tablet(s).

9. You must administer 1250 mg of a drug. The tablets available are 0.25 g each. You will give _____ tablet(s).

10. Tablets are available in 0.25 mg form and the order reads: "Administer 500 μgm." How many tablet(s) will you give?

11. Tablets are available in 250 mcg form, and you must administer 0.5 mg. You give _____ tablet(s).

12. A drug comes as 0.5 mg per tablet, and you must administer 0.25 mg. You will give _____ tablet(s).

13. A medicine comes as 0.01 mg per tablet, and you must administer 50 mcg. You will give _____ tablet(s).

14. You must administer 0.625 mg. You have tablets available in the following strengths, in milligrams: 0.6, 0.5, 0.31, 0.25, 0.125, and 0.1. How many tablets of what strength will you use?

15. You must administer 0.5 mg. You have tablets available in the following strengths, in milligrams: 1.0, 0.75, 0.25, 0.2, 0.125, and 0.1. How many tablets of what strength will you give?

16. You must administer 0.25 mg. Indicate how many of the following tablets you would give for this dosage:

Strength	Number of Tablets
(a) 0.5 mg	_____
(b) 0.125 mg	_____

17. You must administer 0.1 mg. Indicate how many of the following tablets you would give for this dosage:

Strength	Number of Tablets
(a) 0.2 mg	_____
(b) 0.05 mg	_____

► Compare your answers with those listed at the end of this chapter. If you have mastered Activity Sheets 4A and 4B with 100% accuracy, proceed to read and memorize the data in the next section. If you did not master these activity sheets, review the previous text and redo the incorrect problems. Then proceed to the next section.

CALCULATING DOSAGES ACCORDING TO KILOGRAMS OF BODY WEIGHT AND DETERMINING IF A PRESCRIBED DOSE LIES WITHIN THE STIPULATED SAFETY RANGE

As you read literature on drugs, you will find that the therapeutic dosage for a drug is frequently stated in terms of the weight of a person; for example, a recommended dose may be 4 mg/kg of body weight. It is unlikely that you will be responsible for prescribing the dose of a drug for a patient but it is necessary for you to understand how to calculate this dose so that you can verify if a prescribed dose corresponds to what the literature recommends.

Example

The literature states a dose for a person should be 6 mg/kg of body weight. The patient weighs 50 kg. How much should this patient receive?

Dosage
  = Body weight in kg × amount of medication per kg of body weight
  = 50 kg × 6 mg/kg = 300 mg

Example

The literature states the usual adult dosage is 7 mg/kg of body weight and a person should not receive more than 550 mg of the drug per day. The patient weighs 60 kg.
The medication order reads:

Drug y 140 mg t.i.d.

Is this a safe drug dosage? Would you administer it?

Recommended Dose of Literature

Dosage
  = Body weight in kg × amount of medication per kg of body weight
  = 60 kg × 7 mg/kg = 420 mg

Dosage Patient Is Receiving

Dosage
  = Amount of medication per dose × number of doses per day
  = 140 mg × 3 = 420 mg

Decision: The dose appears safe—it is the same as the therapeutic dose recommended in the literature and the amount of the three doses together does not exceed the upper limits—550 mg per day.

▶   When you feel confident of the data in this section, do the problems on Activity Sheet 5.

Activity Sheet 5

1. The drug literature states that the recommended loading dose is 7.5 mg/kg of body weight. The patient weighs 65 kg. How many mg should this patient receive?

2. The drug literature states: recommended dose 5 mg/kg/day in 3 or 4 divided doses. The drug order for this 75 kg person is 125 mg t.i.d. Does this drug order seem appropriate?

3. The drug literature states: the initial dose is 5 mcg/kg/min. The patient is 73 kg. This means the dose this patient should receive of this drug per minute is _____ mcg.

4. The drug literature reads that the recommended dose is 150 mg/kg/day. The patient is 50 kg and is receiving 2.5 G q 8°. Does this drug order seem appropriate?

5. The drug literature states that the initial dose of this drug should be 0.5 mg/kg/day. The patient is 68 kg. How many mg should this person receive per day?

6. The drug literature reads that the recommended dose is 40 mcg/kg/minute. The patient weighs 65 kg. The patient, therefore, should receive _____ mg per minute.

7. The drug literature states that the therapeutic dose of a drug for a 40-kg person is 22.5 mg of that drug per kg of their body weight. This means the person should receive _____ g.

8. The drug literature states that the maximum dose is 50 mcg/kg/min. The patient is 70 kg. This means the most this person can receive of this drug per minute is _____ mg.

9. The drug literature gives the recommended dose as 30 mg/kg/day given in two divided dosages. The person is 55 kg. You would, therefore, expect the order to be _____ mg b.i.d.

10. The drug literature recommends 200 mg/kg/day divided and given in 6 to 8 doses per day. The patient weighs 90 kg. You would expect the prescribed order to read _____ g q 4°.

▶   Compare your answers with those listed at the end of this chapter. If you have answered the questions in Activity Sheet 5 with 100% accuracy proceed to read and memorize the data in the next section. If you did not master this activity sheet, review the previous text and redo the incorrect problems. Then proceed to the next section.

DETERMINING AND READING FLUID VOLUMES OF DOSAGES MEASURED IN A MEDICATION CUP

You have already calculated dosage problems that are similar to the ones contained in this section. The aspect that is added here is practice in your ability to decide the appropriate amount of fluid volume to be prepared in a medication cup in order to administer the prescribed calculated dosage.

Example

Dosage ordered: 375 mg of medication t.i.d.
The medication is available as 125 mg/5 cc.
Decide the fluid volume to give the prescribed dose.

Ratio–Proportion Method

Dose on hand   Desired dose

$$\frac{125 \text{ mg}}{5 \text{ cc}} = \frac{375 \text{ mg}}{x \text{ (cc)}}$$

$$125 \, x = 375 \times 5$$

$$125x = 1875$$

$$x = 15 \text{ cc}$$

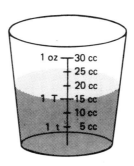

Prescribed dose 15 cc contains 375 mg.

Formula Method

$$\text{Dose} = \frac{\text{Desired dose}}{\text{Dose on hand}} \times \text{amount of vehicle per dose on hand}$$

$$\text{Dose} = \frac{375 \text{ mg}}{125 \text{ mg}} \times 5 \text{ cc}$$

$$= \frac{\overset{3}{\cancel{375}}}{\underset{1}{\cancel{125}}} \times 5 = 15 \text{ cc}$$

▶   When you feel confident of the data in this section, do the problems on Activity Sheet 6.

Activity Sheet 6

For the following problems draw a medication cup and shade in the amount of fluid volume you would pour into the cup to administer the prescribed dose.

    1. Dosage ordered: 1 g
       Dose on hand: 500 mg per 5 cc

    2. Dosage ordered: 0.5 g
       Dose on hand: 250 mg per 5 cc

    3. Prescribed dose: 375 mg
       Dose on hand: 125 mg per 5 cc

    4. Prescribed dose: 0.25 g
       Dose on hand: 125 mg per 5 cc

    5. Prescribed dose: 30 cc

For the following problems (a) calculate the amount of medication the person should receive and (b) draw a medication cup and shade in the amount of fluid volume you would pour into the cup to administer the prescribed dose.

6. Drug literature states the recommended dosage for a medication is 45 mg/kg/day. The person weighs 25 kg. The medication is available as 225 mg per 5 cc.

7. Drug information recommends: 30 mg/kg/day in two divided doses.
   Drug is available as: 125 mg per 5 cc
   Patient weighs: 25 kg

8. Drug literature recommends: 40 mg/kg/day
   Drug is available as: 400 mg per 5 cc
   Patient weighs: 40 kg

9. Drug information recommends: 30 mg/kg/day in two divided doses
   Drug is available as: 250 mg per 5 cc
   Patient weighs: 50 kg

10. Drug literature recommends: 50 mg/kg/day
    Drug is available as: 0.4 g per 5 cc
    Patient weighs: 80 kg

▶ Compare your answers with those listed at the end of this chapter. If you have answered the questions in Activity Sheet 6 with 100% accuracy proceed to read and memorize the data in the next section. If you did not master this activity sheet, review the previous text and redo the incorrect problems. Then proceed to the next section.

MEASUREMENT OF FLUID VOLUME IN A SYRINGE

After completing the previous sections you should feel confident regarding the mathematical process of calculating the dosages of the following problems. This section's focus, however, will go a step beyond this point. It was developed to verify your accuracy in regards to the drawing up of the fluid volume to administer that prescribed calculated dose.

Example

A medication comes as

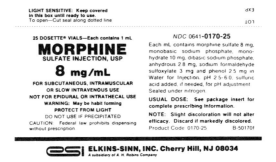

and you must administer 2 mg. How much fluid volume will you draw up into the syringe to administer this dose? Shade in the amount on the syringe. (Remember: Your answer can be expressed in either cc or mL, as they are equivalent.)

Ratio–Proportion Method

$$\text{Dose on hand} = \text{Desired dose}$$

$$\frac{8 \text{ mg}}{1 \text{ cc}} = \frac{2 \text{ mg}}{x \text{ cc}}$$

$$8x = 2$$

$$x = \frac{2}{8} = \frac{1}{4} = 0.25 \text{ cc (mL)}$$

Formula Method

$$\text{Dose} = \frac{\text{Desired dose}}{\text{Dose on hand}} \times \text{amount of vehicle per dose on hand}$$

$$= \frac{2 \text{ mg}}{8 \text{ mg}} \times 1 \text{ cc}$$

$$= \frac{2}{8} \times 1 = \frac{1}{4} = 0.25 \text{ mL (cc)}$$

After calculating the fluid volume to administer you must select a syringe on which you can measure it. Although syringes come in many varied sizes, diagramed below are only the syringes you will most frequently be using.

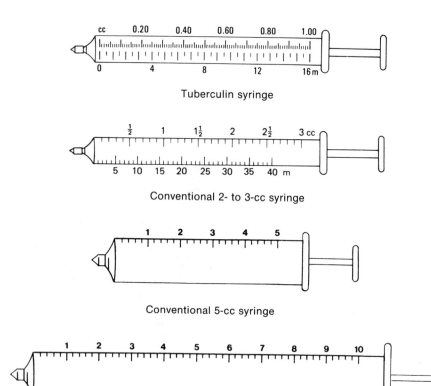

Tuberculin syringe

Conventional 2- to 3-cc syringe

Conventional 5-cc syringe

Conventional 10-cc syringe

(Another common syringe—the insulin syringe—is discussed in Chapter 5.)

You will note that the calibrations on the various syringes are different. Therefore, you must be careful in your selection of a syringe to measure the fluid volume you want to administer. For the example problem you would select the tuberculin syringe because it is calibrated for a measurement of 0.25 cc.

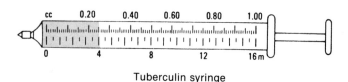

Tuberculin syringe

MEASUREMENT OF FLUID VOLUMES THAT ARE LESS THAN 1 CC

For the measurement of very small volumes of medicated fluid for injection, a tuberculin syringe, shown in the figure below is frequently better than the conventional 2- to 3-cc syringe. Because it is a long, slender syringe, there is more space between each calibration, making it a finer instrument of measurement.

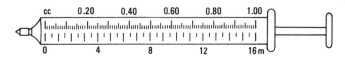

Tuberculin syringe

A tuberculin syringe is safer and more accurate for administering fluid volume measured in tenths of a cubic centimeter. It can also accurately measure such doses as 0.25 cc or 0.75 cc. These doses could not be measured on the conventional 2- to 3-cc syringe, shown below, for the smallest calibrations on this syringe are tenths of a cubic centimeter. These doses would have to be converted and measured utilizing the apothecary measurement of minims. (See Chapter 15.)

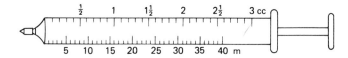

Conventional 2- to 3-cc syringe

▶   When you feel confident of the data in this section, do the problems on Activity Sheet 7.

Activity Sheet 7

For the following four problems place an arrow indicating the accurate calibration line on the syringe that corresponds to the fluid volume you must administer:

1. 1.6 cc

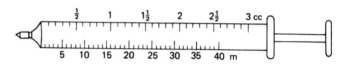

Conventional 2- to 3-cc syringe

2. 0.66 cc

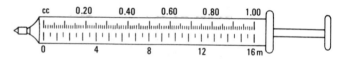

Tuberculin syringe

3. 3.2 cc

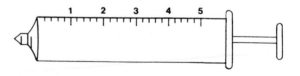

Conventional 5-cc syringe

4. 5.6 cc

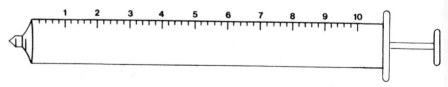

Conventional 10-cc syringe

5. When might you use a tuberculin syringe for measuring fluid for injection?

6. What are the benefits of using a tuberculin syringe to measure a dosage?

7. Using the conventional 2- to 3-cc syringe, how could you measure 0.75 (3/4) cc of fluid?

For problems 8 through 15 calculate the fluid volume you would administer, draw and label the syringe you would use to administer it, and draw an arrow pointing to the calibration line that indicates the amount you should give.

8. Dose on hand: 0.5 mg per 2 cc
   Desired dose: 0.25 mg

9. Dose on hand: 80 mg per 2 cc
   Desired dose: 60 mg

10. Dose on hand: 75 mg per 2 cc
    Prescribed dose: 15 mg

11. Dose on hand: 10 mg/cc
    Prescribed dose: 44 mg

12. Dose on hand:

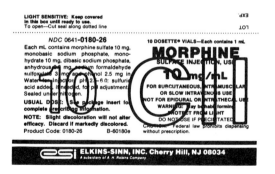

Desired dose: 3 mg

13. Dose on hand: 75 mg per 2 cc
    Prescribed dose: 67.5 mg

14. Dose on hand: 1 g per 3 cc
    Prescribed dose: 250 mg

15. Dose on hand: 0.5 mg per 2 cc
    Desired dose: 0.125 mg

▶ Compare your answers with those listed at the end of this chapter. If you have answered the questions in Activity Sheet 7 with 100% accuracy, proceed to read and memorize the data in the next section. If you did not master this activity sheet, review the previous text and redo the incorrect problems. Then proceed to the next section.

PREPARING MEDICATIONS FROM POWDERED FORM

Many medications for parenteral administration are available in a powdered form and contained in sterile devices such as a vial or an ampule, shown in the accompanying figures:

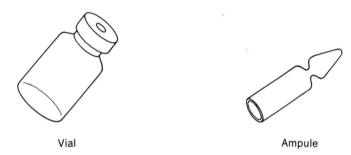

Vial   Ampule

Before administering such medications, it is often your responsibility to reconstitute it to a liquid form. Literature usually accompanies the product and contains the directions for reconstitution. The three most common sterile solutions required as diluents are sterile water for injection, sterile normal saline for injection, and a specific sterile diluent that accompanies the medication. For the intravenous administration of medications, you may find suggested that certain prepared intravenous solutions such as 5% dextrose in water (D_5W) may be used as the diluting agent.

In reconstituting the solution you must keep certain facts in mind: (1) The more dilute the solution, the less irritating it is to tissue and the more rapidly it will be absorbed and act. (2) The usual amount of fluid volume administered intramuscularly is 1 to 2 cc. (3) The usual amount of fluid volume administered subcutaneously is up to 1 cc. Your aim, therefore, is to administer a prescribed dose in as dilute a concentration as can be prepared while remaining within the parameters of the usual amount of fluid volume that is administered via the ordered route. The specifics with regard to fluid volume and medications administered via the intravenous route are discussed in another chapter.

Solution Preparation

To prepare the solution, follow the steps below:

1. Read the available literature (sometimes the same literature and dilution table are used for varied strengths of the medication).
2. Select a package of appropriate medication that contains a dose level closest to the one ordered.
3. Select the type of solution to be used for a diluent.
4. Survey the dilution table and determine the selection that re-

constitutes the solution to the concentration that meets the parameters previously stated.

5. Add the recommended type and amount of fluid volume to the powdered medication.

6. Be sure that all the powdered particles of medication dissolve and the solution becomes completely clear and free of bubbles before it is aspirated into the syringe. (You may need to shake or roll the medication container in your hands to facilitate the dissolving of the powder.)

7. Label the bottle if it contains additional doses; include the
   (a) dilution strength,
   (b) date and time of reconstitution,
   (c) date and time of expiration, and
   (d) preparer's initials

8. Store the medication appropriately. Many medications must be refrigerated, some have to be stored away from direct light, and so on.

Example

Prescribed dose: 250 mg IM (intramuscularly)

Packages of medication available: 125 mg, 250 mg, 500 mg, and 1 g.

To solve, follow the steps listed below:

1,2. Accompanying literature reviewed (see Directions below) and the package of medication selected (250 mg).

DIRECTIONS

1. Use sterile normal saline as the diluent.
2. Follow the dilution table below.
3. Shake the container to facilitate dissolving.
4. Store in refrigerator and use within 24 hr after preparation.

Active Ingredient in Container	Recommended Amount of Diluent to Add	Total Fluid Volume	Concentration
(a) 250 mg	1.5 cc	2 cc	125 mg/cc
(b) 250 mg	4.5 cc	5 cc	50 mg/cc
(c) 250 mg	9.5 cc	10 cc	25 mg/cc

3. Sterile normal saline for injection to be used as the diluent.
4. Line (a) selected from the dilution table as the dilution factor to follow.
5. 1.5 cc sterile normal saline for injection added to the powder.
6. (a) Container shaken, solution clear and free of bubbles.
   (b) 2 cc of fluid aspirated and to be administered for the 250-mg prescribed dose.
7. If additional doses were left, the label should include the following information:
   (a) Concentration strength: 125 mg/cc.
   (b) Prepared: Dec. 24, 1988 at 12 AM, GM (initials).
   (c) Expiration date and time: 24 hr after preparation—Dec. 25, 1988 at 12 AM.
8. Store in refrigerator.

▶ When you feel confident of this material, complete Activity Sheet 8.

Activity Sheet 8

1. The average amount of a fluid given in an intramuscular injection is _____ cc.

2. The average amount of fluid given in a subcutaneous injection is _____ cc.

3. Mark T if the statement is true, F if it is false.
   _____ (a) The more diluted a prescribed medication is made, the less irritating it is to tissue.
   _____ (b) The more diluted a medication is made, the faster it will be absorbed.
   _____ (c) The more diluted a prescribed medication dosage is made, the slower it will act.

4. Name the three solutions that are commonly cited as the appropriate diluents for injectable medications.

5. What other solutions may be suggested as diluent agents for certain powdered medications?

6. List the eight steps to follow in the process of preparing a solution (a directional circular is enclosed with the medication).

DIRECTIONS

1. Use sterile normal saline for injection as the diluent.
2. Follow the dilution table below.
3. Use this medication within 12 hours after it is prepared into a solution.

Active Ingredient in Container	Recommended Amount of Diluent to Add	Total Fluid Volume	Concentration
(a) 125 mg	0.8 cc	1 cc	125 mg/cc
(b) 250 mg	1.8 cc	2 cc	125 mg/cc
(c) 500 mg	1.6 cc	2 cc	250 mg/cc
(d) 1 g	1.2 cc	2 cc	500 mg/cc
(e) 1 g	4.4 cc	5 cc	200 mg/cc

For questions 7 through 10 apply the eight steps you listed in answering question 6. For questions 7 and 8 use Directions on p. 94.

7. Prescribed dose: 250 mg IM
   Packages of medication available: 125 mg, 250 mg, 500 mg, and 1 g
   Reference literature available: See p. 94.

8. Prescribed dose: 500 mg IM
   Packages of medication available: 125 mg, 250 mg, 500 mg, and 1 g
   Reference literature available: See p. 94.

9. Prescribed dose: 1000 mg IM
   Packages available: 0.5 g, 1 g, and 2 g
   Reference literature available:

DIRECTIONS

1. Use the enclosed diluent.
2. Follow the dilution table below.
3. Shake the container to facilitate dissolving of the powder.
4. Expires 1 week after being dissolved.
5. Store in a dark area away from direct light.

Active Ingredient in Container	Recommended Amount of Diluent to Add	Total Fluid Volume	Concentration
(a) 500 mg	0.8 cc	1 cc	500 mg/cc
(b) 1 g	1.4 cc	2 cc	500 mg/cc
(c) 1 g	3.4 cc	4 cc	250 mg/cc
(d) 2 g	3.4 cc	4 cc	500 mg/cc
(e) 2 g	1.8 cc	2 cc	1 g/cc

---

10. Prescribed dose: 2 g IM
    Use the reference literature available in question 9.

▶ Compare your answers with those listed at the end of this chapter. If you have mastered these items and all the previous work in this chapter, you are ready to complete the posttest of this chapter. If you have not mastered this material, review the previous text and then correct your mistakes. After this you should be ready for the posttest.

Posttest

1. List the basic units and subunits of the metric system for both liquid measures and measures of weight used in dosage calculations.

2. Write the meaning or give the abbreviation for the following:
    (a) Liter = _____
    (b) Milliliter = _____
    (c) _____ = cc

3. Equivalents:
    (a) 1 mL   = _____ cc   (b) 1000 mL   = _____ L
    (c) 1 L   = _____ cc   (d) 1000 cc   = _____ L
    (e) 1 L   = _____ mL   (f) 1 cc   = _____ mL

4. (a) State the rule to convert liters to milliliters.
    (b) State the rule to convert milliliters to liters.

5. Convert:
    (a) 3.0 L   = _____ mL   (b) 300 mL   = _____ L
    (c) 4.75 L   = _____ cc   (d) 2040 cc   = _____ L
    (e) 630 cc   = _____ L   (f) 1.3 L   = _____ cc
    (g) 2500 mL   = _____ L   (h) 2.05 L   = _____ mL

6. Add:
    (a) 6 L + 30 cc + 250 mL + 4.5 L + 0.4 L = _____ L
    (b) 3 L + 75 cc + 125 cc + 2.75 L + 0.25 L = _____ cc

7. (a) State the rule to convert grams to milligrams.
    (b) State the rule to convert milligrams to grams.
    (c) State the rule to convert milligrams to micrograms.
    (d) State the rule to convert micrograms to milligrams.

8. Convert:
    (a) 1000 mg   = _____ g   (b) 0.5 g   = _____ mg
    (c) 2.35 g   = _____ mg   (d) 630 mg   = _____ g
    (e) 1 mg   = _____ g   (f) 1.8 g   = _____ mg
    (g) 330 mg   = _____ g   (h) 0.9 g   = _____ mg

TPO	IPO	
	16,18	9. Convert:

9. Convert:

   (a) 1 mg   = _____ mcg   (b) 0.325 mg = _____ mcg
   (c) 650 mcg = _____ mg   (d) 0.06 mg   = _____ mcg
   (e) 550 mcg = _____ mg   (f) 0.1 mg   = _____ mcg
   (g) 0.125 mg = _____ mcg   (h) 3000 mcg = _____ mg

21

10. From the following list identify the active ingredient (the medication component) as opposed to the vehicle that carries it:
   (a) 4.0 g per 4 cc   (b) 50 g per 250 cc
   (c) one capsule is 40 mcg   (d) 1 cc contains 400 mg
   (e) 0.1 mg per tablet

1   19

11. A medication is available as 0.5 g/cc and you must administer 0.125 g. You will give _____ cc. (To calculate, use the ratio–proportion method.)

1   19

12. A medication is available as 0.1 g per tablet and you must administer 0.05 g. You will give _____ tablet(s). (To calculate, use the ratio–proportion method.)

2   20

13. A medication is available as 0.75 g per 1.5 cc and you must administer 0.25 g. You will give _____ cc. (To calculate, use the formula method.)

1   20

14. A medication is available as 0.25 g per tablet and you must administer 0.5 g. You will give _____ tablet(s). (To calculate, use the formula method.)

3   19 or 20

15. A drug is available as 500 mg/cc and you must administer 0.375 g. You will give _____ cc.

2   19 or 20

16. A drug is available as 0.6 g per tablet and you must administer 300 mg. You will give _____ tablet(s).

3   19 or 20

17. A drug is available as 0.75 g per cc and you must have 900 mg. You will give _____ cc.

3   19 or 20

18. A medicine is available as 0.5 g/L. How many milligrams are there in 1 cc?

6   19

19. A medicine is available as 0.75 g per 1.5 L. You must administer 5 mg. How many cubic centimeters is this?

7,9,10

20. A patient's fluid intake consists of breakfast 0.52 L, lunch 325 cc, dinner 635 mL, and in-between feedings 0.4 L. What is his total fluid intake in cc?

TPO	IPO	
2	19 or 20	21. You must administer 0.25 g. The medication is available as 125 mg per tablet. You will administer _____ tablet(s).
4	19 or 20	22. A doctor's order reads: "Administer 0.5 mg by mouth." The liquid preparation is 125 mcg per 5 cc. You will give _____ cc.
4	19 or 20	23. The physician orders 100 mcg in a liquid preparation to be taken by mouth. The solution is available as 0.05 mg per 5 cc. You will give _____ cc.
5	19 or 20	24. You must administer 0.375 mg. The following tablets are available: 0.125 mg, 0.25 mg, 0.5 mg, 0.75 mg, and 3.75 mg. You should administer _____ .
5	19 or 20	25. You must administer 0.75 g. The following oral liquid solutions are available: 7.5 mg/cc, 25 mg per 5 cc, 50 mg per 5 cc, and 75 mg/cc. You should administer _____ .
7		26. Drug literature states that the recommended dose is 7 mg/kg of body weight. The patient weighs 68 kg. How many mg should he receive?
7	15,16	27. Drug data state that the recommended dose is 20 mcg/kg of body weight. The patient weighs 80 kg. The patient must receive _____ mg.
8		28. A recommended drug dose is 5 mg/kg of body weight in four equally divided doses. The patient weighs 100 kg. The prescribed order reads for you to administer 125 mg q.i.d. Does this order seem appropriate?
8		29. A recommended dose is 150 mg/kg/day. The patient weighs 65 kg and is receiving 3.25 g q 8°. Does this order seem appropriate?
9	11,19, or 20	30. A drug is available as 250 mg per 5 cc and you must administer 0.75 g. Draw an arrow to indicate the amount of fluid volume you would pour into this cup to administer this dosage.

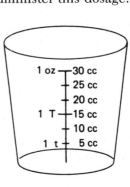

TPO   IPO
9   22,23

31. A drug is available as 8 mg/cc and you must administer 6 mg. Draw the type syringe you would use and place an arrow to indicate the amount of fluid volume you would prepare in the syringe to administer this dose.

10   24–30

32. Prescribed dose: 250 mg IM. In reference to the directions below, answer the following:
    (a) What diluent should be used?
    (b) What dilution strength would you select?
    (c) How much fluid volume would you administer intramuscularly?
    (d) What would you write on the bottle label after you have prepared this?

DIRECTIONS

1. Use sterile water for injection as the diluent.
2. Follow the dilution table below.
3. Use within 24 hours after reconstitution.

Active Ingredient in Container	Recommended Amount of Diluent to Add	Total Fluid Volume	Concentration
(a) 1 g	1.8 cc	2 cc	500 mg/cc
(b) 2 g	6.6 cc	8 cc	500 mg/2 cc
(c) 500 mg	3.4 cc	4 cc	250 mg/2 cc
(d) 250 mg	0.9 cc	1 cc	250 mg/cc
(e) 125 mg	0.5 cc	1 cc	125 mg/cc

► Turn to the end of the chapter to check your answers. If you have mastered this test, begin the next chapter. If you have not mastered this test, note the number of the objective next to each incorrect test item. Return to the text related to this objective. Review it. Redo some problems on the previous activity sheets that are similar to the ones you did incorrectly on this posttest and then redo the incorrect test items here. After this you should be ready to take the pretest of this chapter as a second posttest. Correct it, review it, and then continue on to the next chapter.

Answers for Chapter 4

PRETEST

1. Liquid measures: basic unit—liter; subunit—cubic centimeter or milliliter.
   Weight: basic unit—gram; subunits—milligram and microgram.
2. (a) L, l   (b) cc   (c) Milliliter
3. (a) 1   (b) 1000   (c) 1000   (d) 1   (e) 1   (f) 1
4. (a) To convert liters to milliliters multiply by 1000
   (b) To convert milliliters to liters divide by 1000
5. (a) 4000   (b) 0.4   (c) 6750   (d) 3.05   (e) 0.52
   (f) 1700   (g) 3   (h) 2050
6. (a) 9120   (b) 9.13
7. (a) To convert grams to milligrams, multiply by 1000
   (b) To convert milligrams to grams, divide by 1000
   (c) To convert milligrams to micrograms, multiply by 1000
   (d) To convert micrograms to milligrams, divide by 1000
8. (a) 1000   (b) 0.5   (c) 1250   (d) 0.65   (e) 0.001
   (f) 1700   (g) 0.74   (h) 300
9. (a) 1000   (b) 275   (c) 0.45   (d) 30   (e) 0.3
   (f) 800   (g) 375   (h) 4

10.

Active Ingredient	Vehicle
(a) 10 mcg	1 tablet
(b) 500 mg	5 cc
(c) 60 g	500 cc
(d) 250 mcg	1 capsule
(e) 1 g	1 cc

11. 1.25   12. 2   13. 0.5

14. 0.5   15. 0.5   16. 2

17. 0.5   18. 250   19. 4

20. 0.56   21. 2   22. 25

23. 25

24. Two 0.25. It is best to give (a) fewest number of tablets and (b) tablets that are not split.

25. 25 cc of the 125 mg/5 cc. It is best to give volume of between 5 and 30 cc for an oral liquid preparation.

26. 396
27. 2.25
28. Yes. The person is to receive 400 mg/day. An order of 100 mg 4 times a day would be equal to this.
29. Yes. The person is to receive 11,250 mg/day. Three doses (one every 8 hr) of 3750 mg (3.75 g) would equal this.
30.

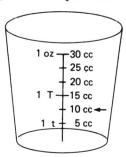

31. Diagram tuberculin syringe arrow to 0.7 cc.

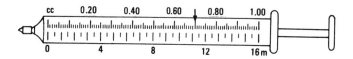

32. (a) Normal saline for injection
    (b) 50 mg/cc
    (c) 2 cc
    (d) (1) Concentration strength 50 mg/cc
        (2) Date and time prepared
        (3) Date and time expires
        (4) Preparer's initials

ACTIVITY SHEET 1

1. The metric system
2. Smaller
3. Weight and volume
4. Metric
5. Metric
6. Decimals
7. The substance that causes a drug to act
8. The substance that carries or contains the active ingredient
9. Gram, milligram, microgram

10. Liter, milliliter, cubic centimeter
11. Capsules, tablets, spansules
12.

Active Ingredient	Vehicle
(a) 0.4 mg	1 mL
(b) 10 mg	1 mL
(c) 15 mg	1 mL

13. Consider:
    (a) Do not give split tablets if this can be avoided.
    (b) Give the fewest number of tablets.
14. (a) 5 to 30 cc
    (b) Up to 3 cc (1 to 2 being the most common)
    (c) 1 cc or below

ACTIVITY SHEET 2

1. Liter
2. Cubic centimeter or milliliter
3. (a) mL   (b) Cubic centimeter   (c) L, l
4. (a) 1000   (b) 1
5. To convert liters to milliliters or cubic centimeters, multiply by 1000.
6. (a) 2000   (b) 300   (c) 120   (d) 3620   (e) 1300
   (f) 2400   (g) 9   (h) 5000   (i) 150   (j) 500
7. To convert milliliters to liters, divide by 1000.
8. (a) 0.325   (b) 0.05   (c) 2.5   (d) 0.175   (e) 3.02
   (f) 0.25   (g) 3.6   (h) 4.57   (i) 0.075   (j) 0.75
9. 2.5
10. (a) 1600   (b) 1.6
11. 2.75
12. 3500
13. 1925
14. 2.5
15. 2250

ACTIVITY SHEET 3

1. Gram
2. Milligram and microgram
3. (a) Gram   (b) Microgram   (c) Milligram
   (d) mcg, μg, mcgm, μgm (e) g, gm, G, Gm   (f) mg, mgm
4. (a) 1000   (b) 1000   (c) 1   (d) 1

5. To convert grams to milligrams, multiply by 1000.
6. To convert milligrams to grams, divide by 1000.
7. (a) 0.1   (b) 0.01   (c) 1.5   (d) 6   (e) 65   (f) 50
    (g) 0.03   (h) 0.85   (i) 0.004   (j) 0.25   (k) 0.75   (l) 1700
    (m) 3620   (n) 1
8. To convert milligrams to micrograms, multiply by 1000.
9. To convert micrograms to milligrams, divide by 1000.
10. (a) 0.15   (b) 0.8   (c) 900   (d) 125   (e) 5   (f) 375
    (g) 0.25   (h) 50   (i) 0.405   (j) 1

ACTIVITY SHEET 4A

1. 5   2. 20   3. 2
4. 1.5   5. 0.5   6. 2.5
7. 2   8. 9   9. 1.5
10. 0.75 cc   11. 2.5 cc   12. 1.25 cc
13. 0.5 cc   14. 4 cc   15. 1.5
16. 1
17. (a) 0.8   (b) 0.6
18. (a) 0.7   (b) 1.25

ACTIVITY SHEET 4B

1. (a) 4   (b) 2   2. 0.5   3. 0.5
4. 3   5. 2   6. 2
7. 2   8. 0.5   9. 5
10. 2   11. 2   12. 0.5
13. 5
14. One 0.5 and one 0.125
15. Two 0.25
16. (a) One-half 0.5   (b) Two 0.125
17. (a) One-half 0.2   (b) Two 0.05

ACTIVITY SHEET 5

1. 487.5
2. Yes. The total dose the person should receive is 375 mg, and 125 mg three times a day equal this.
3. 365

4. Yes. The total dose this person should receive is 7500 mg (7.5 g) and 2.5 G q 8° (i.e., three times a day) equals this.
5. 34
6. 2.6
7. 0.9
8. 3.5
9. 825
10. 3

ACTIVITY SHEET 6

1. 10 cc

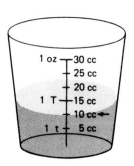

2. 10 cc

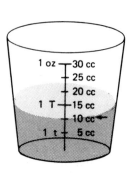

3. 15 cc

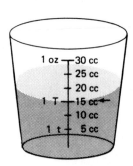

4. 10 cc

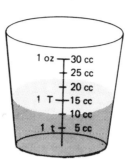

5. 30 cc

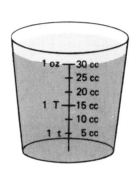

6. (a) 1125 mg/day
   (b) 25 cc

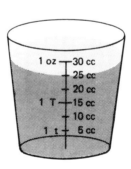

7. (a) 2 doses of 375 mg each
   (b) 15 cc (each dose)

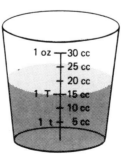

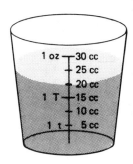

8. (a) 1600 mg/day
   (b) 20 cc

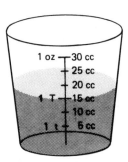

9. (a) 2 doses 750 mg each
   (b) 15 cc (each dose)

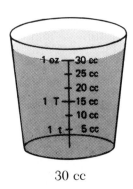 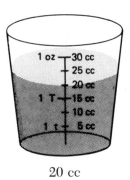

10. (a) 4000 mg
    (b) 50 cc total

30 cc   20 cc

ACTIVITY SHEET 7

1. Diagram a 2- to 3-cc syringe. Arrow to 1.6 cc.

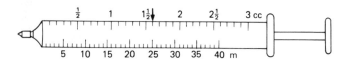

2. Diagram tuberculin syringe. Arrow to 0.66 cc.

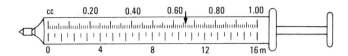

3. Diagram 5-cc syringe. Arrow to 3.2 cc.

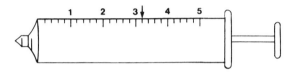

4. Diagram 10-cc syringe. Arrow to 5.6 cc.

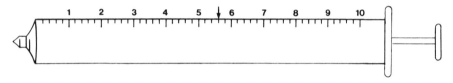

5. To administer small volumes of medication (less than 1 cc), particularly when measured in tenths of a cubic centimeter, or such volumes as 0.25 cc.

6. It provides increased safety and accuracy for measuring small volumes. It provides a means to measure certain volumes accurately without conversion, which could not be done on a conventional 2- to 3-cc syringe.

7. You would have to convert it to the apothecary system and measure it using the other scale on the syringe.

8. 1 cc. Picture: Tuberculin syringe or 2- to 3-cc syringe.

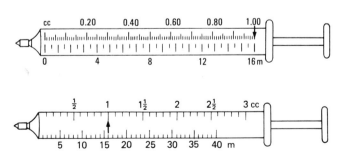

9. 1½ cc. Diagram 2- to 3-cc syringe.

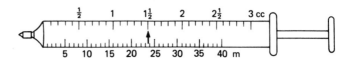

10. 0.4 cc. Diagram tuberculin syringe.

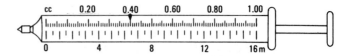

11. 4.4 cc. Diagram 5-cc syringe.

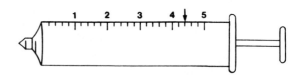

12. 0.3 cc. Tuberculin syringe diagram.

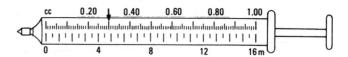

13. 1.8 cc. Diagram 2- to 3-cc syringe.

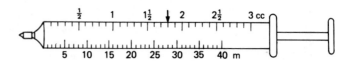

14. 0.75 cc. Diagram tuberculin syringe.

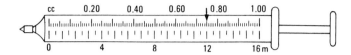

15. 0.5 cc. Diagram tuberculin syringe.

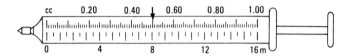

ACTIVITY SHEET 8

1. 1 to 2
2. up to 1
3. (a) T   (b) T   (c) F
4. (a) Sterile water for injection
   (b) Sterile normal saline for injection
   (c) A specific sterile diluent that accompanies the powdered medication
5. Certain commercially prepared intravenous solutions such as 5% dextrose in water
6. Please check the list located in the section of text of this chapter entitled Preparing Medications from Powdered Form.
7. *Steps 1 and 2:* Literature reviewed, package selected: 250 mg for IM use.
   Step 3: Sterile normal saline for injection selected as the diluent.
   Step 4: (b) is selected from dilution table as the dilution factor to follow; gives the prescribed dose in the best concentration.
   Step 5: 1.8 cc sterile normal saline added to container.
   Step 6: (a) Solution clear and free of bubbles. (b) 2 cc of fluid aspirated and to be administered for the 250 mg dose.
   Step 7: If additional doses were left, label should read: "125 mg/cc, prepared Dec. 25, 1987, at 12 AM, GM (initials). Expires Dec. 25, 1987, at 12 PM" (12 hr after dilution). (The preparation and expiration dates and times, and the preparer's initials vary, of course, to suit the specific circumstances.)
   Step 8: No special storage information noted.
8. *Steps 1 and 2:* Literature reviewed and 1-g package selected.
   Step 3: Sterile normal saline for injection used as diluent.

Step 4: (c) selected from dilution table as the dilution factor to follow; gives the prescribed dose in the best concentration.

Step 5: 1.6 cc sterile normal saline added.

Step 6: (a) Solution clear and free of bubbles. (b) 2 cc of fluid aspirated and to be administered for the 500 mg dose.

Step 7: Additional doses are left. Label should read: "250 mg/cc prepared Dec. 25, 1987, at 12 AM, GM (initials). Expires Dec. 25, 1987, at 12 PM" (12 hr after dilution). (The preparation and expiration dates and times, and the preparer's initials vary, of course, to suit the specific circumstances.)

Step 8: No special storage indicated.

9. *Steps 1 and 2:* Literature reviewed. Package selected. The 1-g or the 2-g dose might be appropriate. If this is a one-time dose, then the 1-g package is the best to select. There will be no waste, for the medication lasts only 1 week. If this medication is to be given again within the day or week, mixing the 2-g container will leave a subsequent dose ready for the next time it is to be administered.

Step 3: The special enclosed diluent is used.

Step 4: If the 1-g package is used, (b) is the selection from the dilution table that should be followed. If the 2-g package is used, (d) is the selection from the dilution table that should be followed.

Step 5: For the 1-g package, add 1.4 cc of the special diluent to the container. For the 2-g package, add 3.4 cc of the special diluent to the container.

Step 6: (a) The container is shaken to facilitate dissolving of the powder. (b) 2 cc of fluid is aspirated and administered for a 1-g prescribed dose.

Step 7: For the 2-g container: additional doses are left. The label should read: "500 mg/cc, prepared Dec. 25, 1987, at 1 AM, GM (initials). Expires Jan. 1, 1988, at 1 AM" (1 week after dilution). (The preparation and expiration dates and times, and the preparer's initials vary, of course, to suit the specific circumstances.)

Step 8: Store in a dark area away from direct light.

10. *Steps 1 and 2:* Literature reviewed and the 2-g package selected.

Step 3: Special enclosed diluent utilized.

Step 4: (e) is selected from the dilution tables as the dilution factor to follow.

Step 5: 1.8 cc of special diluent added to the container.

Step 6: (a) The container is shaken to facilitate dissolving of the powder. (b) 2 cc of fluid is aspirated and to be administered for a 2-g prescribed dose.

Step 7: If additional doses were available the label should read: "1 g/cc, prepared Dec. 25, 1987 at 1 AM Expires Jan. 1, 1988 at 1 AM (1 week after dilution), GM (initials)."

Step 8: Storage should be in a darkened area away from direct light.

POSTTEST

1. Liquid measures; basic unit—liter; subunit—cubic centimeter or milliliter.
   Weight: basic unit—gram; subunits—milligram and microgram.
2. (a) L, l   (b) mL, ml   (c) cubic centimeter
3. (a) 1   (b) 1   (c) 1000   (d) 1   (e) 1000   (f) 1
4. (a) To convert liters to milliliters multiply by 1000.
   (b) To convert milliliters to liters divide by 1000.
5. (a) 3000   (b) 0.3   (c) 4750   (d) 2.04   (e) 0.63
   (f) 1300   (g) 2.5   (h) 2050
6. (a) 11.18   (b) 6200
7. (a) To convert grams to milligrams, multiply by 1000.
   (b) To convert milligrams to grams, divide by 1000.
   (c) To convert milligrams to micrograms, multiply by 1000.
   (d) To convert micrograms to milligrams, divide by 1000.
8. (a) 1   (b) 500   (c) 2350   (d) 0.63   (e) 0.001
   (f) 1800   (g) 0.33   (h) 900
9. (a) 1000   (b) 325   (c) 0.65   (d) 60   (e) 0.55
   (f) 100   (g) 125   (h) 3
10.

Active Ingredient	Vehicle
(a) 4 g	4 cc
(b) 50 g	250 cc
(c) 40 mcg	1 capsule
(d) 400 mg	1 cc
(e) 0.1 mg	1 tablet

11. 0.25   12. 0.5   13. 0.5
14. 2   15. 0.75   16. 0.5
17. 1.2   18. 0.5   19. 10
20. 1880   21. 2   22. 20
23. 10
24. One 0.125 and one 0.25. It is best to give (a) the fewest number of tablets and (b) tablets that are not split.
25. 10 cc of the 75 mg/cc. It is best to give a volume of between 5 and 30 cc for an oral liquid preparation.
26. 476
27. 1.6
28. Yes. The patient should receive 500 mg/day, and four equally divided doses would be 125 mg each. This is identical to the ordered dose—125 mg four times a day.
29. Yes. The patient is to receive 9750 mg/day. Three doses per day (which is the same as every 8 hours or q 8°) of 3.25 g (3250 mg) equals 9750 mg.

30. 15 cc

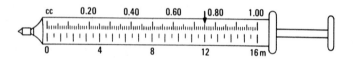

31. Diagram tuberculin syringe. Arrow to 0.75 cc.

32. (a) Sterile water for injection   (b) c   (c) 2 cc
    (d) (1) Concentration 250 mg/2 cc
        (2) Date and time of preparation
        (3) Date and time of expiration
        (4) Preparer's initials

5 | *Other Measurements of Medications*

TERMINAL PERFORMANCE OBJECTIVES

1. Given a prescribed dosage order in units or milliequivalents and the preparation available, the reader is able to calculate the dosage and compute the number of tablets or the amount of fluid volume to be administered.
2. Given an insulin dosage and a diagram of an insulin syringe, the reader is able to mark the calibration line that indicates the accurate amount to be administered.
3. Given a prescribed dosage of U 500 insulin, the reader is able to calculate the amount of fluid volume to prepare for administering the prescribed dose in a tuberculin and a U 100 syringe.

INTERMEDIATE PERFORMANCE OBJECTIVES

After studying the text, the reader is able to do the following:

1. State two common quantities used to measure medicine other than those previously learned in the metric or apothecary systems.
2. Write the abbreviations for the quantities indicated in Intermediate Performance Objective 1.
3. Compute the number of tablets or amount of fluid volume to be administered for a prescribed dosage measured in units or milliequivalents.

4. Explain the meaning of an insulin medication label.
5. State the fact that must be taken into account when an insulin syringe is chosen.

▶   If you feel confident that you have these skills, take the pretest that follows. Otherwise go on to study the data in the first section of this chapter.

Pretest

1. State two commonly used measurements for medications other than those weight measures used in the apothecary or metric system.

2. A drug comes 1,000,000 units (U) per 10 cc and you must administer 300,000 U. You will give _____ cc.

3. A drug comes 5,000,000 U per 25 cc and you must give 500,000 U. You will give _____ cc.

4. A drug comes 10,000,000 U per 20 cc and you must administer 1,250,000 U. You will give _____ cc.

5. A drug is available as 1,000,000 U per 4 cc and you must give 750,000 U. You will give _____ cc.

6. A drug comes 15,000 U/cc and you must give 7,500 U. Indicate the fluid volume you will prepare.

7. A drug comes 40 mEq per 30 cc and you must administer 30 mEq. You will give _____ cc.

8. You must add 4 mEq of a medicine to each liter of fluid. The medication available is 2 mEq/cc. You will add _____ cc to each 2000 cc bottle of fluid.

9. You must add 20 mEq of a drug to 1 L of fluid. The medication is available as 40 mEq per 20 cc. You will use _____ cc of the medication.

10. You must administer 40 mEq of a medicine. It is available as 20 mEq per 15 cc. You will give, therefore, _____ cc.

115

TPO	IPO
1	3

11. You must give 10 mEq of a drug. It is available as 20 mEq per 15 cc. You will give _____ cc.

| 1 | 3 |

12. You must add 40 mEq to each liter of solution. It is available as 2 mEq/cc. You will add _____ cc.

| | 4 |

13. Insulin is labeled U 100; what does this mean?

| | 5 |

14. When you are preparing an insulin dosage, what fact must you take into account as you choose an insulin syringe?

| 2 | |

15. An insulin order is: "8 U of regular insulin and 54 U of a long-acting insulin." Draw an arrow indicating the calibration that is the total amount of insulin that should be prepared. (These two insulins are compatible.)

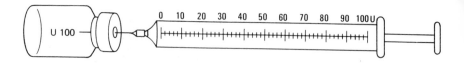

| 2 | |

16. An insulin order is: "6 U of regular insulin and 34 U of a long acting insulin." Draw an arrow indicating the calibration that is the total amount of insulin that should be prepared.

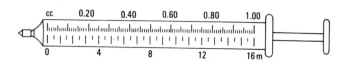

For the following two problems place an arrow indicating the accurate calibration line on the syringe that corresponds to the dose that you must administer.

| 3 | 3 |

17. Administer 425 U of U 500 insulin.

TPO   IPO

3   3   18. Administer 325 U of U 500 insulin.

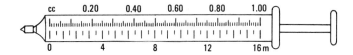

                  For the following prescribed dosages of U 500 insulin calculate the
                  number of units to prepare in a U 100 syringe:

3   3   19. 375 U.

3   3   20. 175 U.

▶   Compare your answers with those listed at the end of this chapter. If you have mastered
     this test, then you may bypass this chapter and begin the next chapter. If you have not
     mastered this test, proceed to memorize the data in the next section on units and
     milliequivalents.

UNITS AND MILLIEQUIVALENTS

Clinically you encounter a number of quantities used in the measurement of medications. Two that you will frequently see are the quantities of units and milliequivalents. As milligrams and grains were quantities to measure the weight of medication, units and milliequivalents also represent a measurement of a given medicine.

No conversion or equivalency exists between units and milliequivalents and the metric and the apothecary systems. Problems containing these quantities are solved relatively easily. You should proceed in the same manner as with your previous calculations.

Abbreviations: unit = U, u; milliequivalent = mEq

Example

There are 10,000 U in 1 cc. The order is to give 7,500 units.

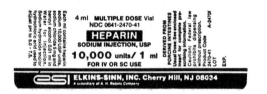

Dose available: 10,000 U/cc
Desired dose: 7,500 U/x cc

Remember, the first ratio is the relationship of the given quantity in the problem; this relates the amount of medication found in the specified vehicle.

$$\text{Dose available} \rightarrow \frac{10,000 \text{ U}}{1 \text{ cc}} = \frac{7,500 \text{ U}}{x} \leftarrow \text{Desired dose}$$
$$\text{Known relationship} \nearrow \qquad \qquad \leftarrow \text{Unknown}$$
$$\text{of quantities}$$

$$10,000\, x = 7,500$$

$$x = \frac{7,500}{10,000}$$

$$x = \frac{3}{4} \text{ or } 0.75 \text{ cc}$$

Example

You must administer 30 mEq. The dose available is

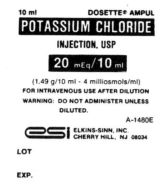

Dose available: 20 mEq/10 mL
Desired dose: 30 mEq/x mL

$$\text{Dose available} \rightarrow \frac{20 \text{ mEq}}{10 \text{ mL}} = \frac{30 \text{ mEq}}{x \text{ mL}} \begin{matrix} \leftarrow \text{Desired dose} \\ \leftarrow \text{Unknown} \end{matrix}$$

Known relationship
of quantities

$$20\, x = 30 \times 10$$

$$20\, x = 300$$

$$x = \frac{300}{20}$$

$$x = 15 \text{ mL}$$

▶   When you feel confident about this material, complete Activity Sheet 1.

Activity Sheet 1

1. State two commonly used measurements for medications, other than those used in the apothecary or metric systems.

2. You must give 500,000 U of a medicine. It is available as 300,000 U/cc. You will give _____ cc.

3. A drug comes 20 mEq per 10 cc and you must give 15 mEq. You will give _____ cc.

4. A drug is available as follows:

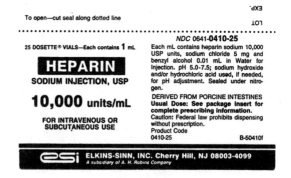

   You must give 30,000 U. Draw a syringe with an arrow indicating the fluid volume you would draw up.

5. You must give 24 mEq. The drug available is 8 mEq per tablet. You will give _____ tablets.

6. A medicine is available as 1,000,000 U in 4 cc and you must administer 500,000 U. You will give _____ cc.

7. A medicine comes as follows:

20 ml   DOSETTE® AMPUL

POTASSIUM CHLORIDE

INJECTION, USP

40 mEq/20 ml

(2.98 g/20 ml - 4 milliosmols/ml)
FOR INTRAVENOUS USE AFTER DILUTION
WARNING: DO NOT ADMINISTER UNLESS
DILUTED.

A-1490D

℮Si | ELKINS-SINN, INC
CHERRY HILL, NJ 08034

LOT

EXP.

You must give 30 mEq. You will give _____ cc.

8. A drug comes as 250,000 U/cc. You must give 750,000 U. You will give _____ cc.

9. A drug is labeled 20 mEq per 15 cc. You must give 30 mEq. You will give _____ cc.

10. A drug is available as 10,000,000 U per 10 cc. You must give 1,500,000 U. You will give _____ cc.

11. A drug comes 1,000,000 U per 5 cc. You must give 600,000 U. You will give _____ cc.

12. A drug is labeled:

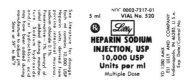

NDC 0002-7217-01
5 ml   VIAL No. 520
℞ | Lilly
HEPARIN SODIUM
INJECTION, USP
10,000 USP
Units per ml
Multiple Dose

You must administer 5000 U. Draw a syringe with an arrow indicating the fluid volume you would draw up.

13. A drug is labeled 10,000,000 U per 20 cc. You must administer 1,000,000 U. You will administer _____ cc.

14. 40 mEq of a medication is ordered. The medicine available is labeled as 20 mEq per 15 cc. You will administer _____ cc.

15. You must add 12 mEq of a drug to every 2 L of solution. The medicine is labeled as 2 mEq/cc. You will add _____ cc.

16. A drug is labeled "40 mEq in each 20 cc vial." You must administer 30 mEq. You will give _____ cc.

17. A drug order is to administer 40 mEq of a drug, three times a day. The solution available is 20 mEq per 15 cc. Therefore you will need _____ cc of this drug for each day.

18. You must add 5 mEq of a drug to each 1000 mL of fluid. The drug is labeled to contain 2 mEq/cc. You will add _____ cc to each liter.

19. A drug is labeled as 40 mEq per 30 cc and you must administer 20 mEq. You will give _____ cc.

20. You must add 3 mEq per 1000 mL. The medication is labeled "2 mEq/cc." How much will be added to a 2-L bottle of fluid?

▶ Compare your answers with those listed at the end of this chapter. If you have mastered these items, proceed on to the text that follows. If you have not mastered this material, review the previous text and then correct your mistakes. After this proceed to the text that follows.

NSULIN ADMINISTRATION

Insulin is an injectable medication that you will frequently administer. It is discussed separately because its labeling and its preparation and administration are somewhat different. It comes labeled as U 500, U 100, and U 40. What this means is that every cubic centimeter of the solution in the multiple-dose bottle contains that stated amount of units of insulin. For example,

U 500 contains 500 units (U) of insulin per cc
U 100 contains 100 U of insulin per cc
U 40 contains 40 U of insulin per cc

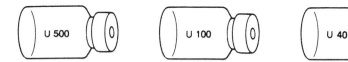

The most common strength that you will use clinically is U 100. This is what we will concentrate on in this section. The administration of U 500 is discussed later. Typical insulin labels are as follows:

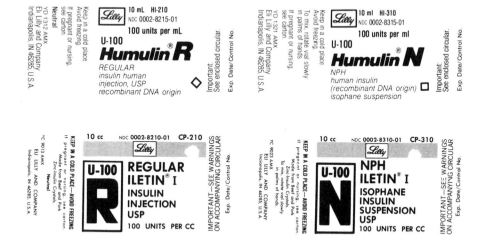

The second most important aspect is that you must use an appropriately calibrated insulin syringe to prepare the dosage for administration. To administer a dosage of U 100 insulin, you must use a syringe calibrated to hold 100 U of insulin and for U 40 insulin a syringe calibrated to hold 40 U of insulin. Both of the syringes shown in the accompanying figure hold only 1 cc of insulin of their respective concentration. These syringes may not be used interchangeably with any other insulin solution. They are intended to hold only the solution concentration for which they were manufactured.

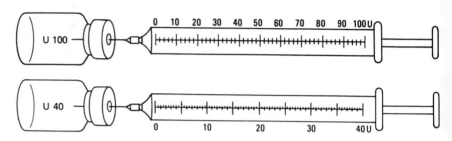

Syringes of 1 cc capacity calibrated for two different concentrations of insulin

INSULIN ADMINISTRATION—A SPECIAL SITUATION

You may occasionally encounter an emergency situation when an insulin syringe is not available and an insulin dose must be administered. To do this you may utilize a tuberculin syringe. The volume of fluid you must draw up into the syringe to administer the prescribed dosage is calculated in the same way you have done other dosage problems. Therefore, you should learn this with relative ease. The following should provide an example and adequate practice to make you feel confident about this skill. Lastly, it must be emphasized that this method should not be common practice. It should be used only in special situations.

Example

Situation: Administer 60 U of insulin—no insulin syringe available.
Identify: Desired dose: 60 U.
 Dose on hand: U 100 (insulin).
Two methods are shown—use the one that is easier for you.

Proportion Method

$$\frac{\text{Dose on hand}}{\text{Vehicle of dose on hand}} = \frac{\text{Desired dose}}{x \text{ (Unknown)}}$$

$$\frac{100 \text{ U}}{1 \text{ cc}} = \frac{60 \text{ U}}{x \text{ (cc)}}$$

$$100x = 60$$

$$x = \frac{60}{100}$$

$$x = \frac{6}{10} \text{ or } 0.6 \text{ cc}$$

Formula Method

$$\text{Dose} = \frac{\text{Desired dose}}{\text{Dose on hand}} \times \text{amount of vehicle per dose on hand}$$

$$= \frac{60 \text{ U}}{100 \text{ U}} \times 1 \text{ cc}$$

$$= \frac{6\cancel{0} \text{ U}}{10\cancel{0} \text{ U}} \times 1 \text{ cc}$$

$$= \frac{6}{10} \times 1 = \frac{6}{10} \text{ or } 0.6 \text{ cc}$$

PREPARATION OF AN INSULIN DOSE

Doctor's order: 40 units of a specific long acting insulin
Possible available insulin: U 100, U 40

To prepare the dosage, fill the syringe with the amount of insulin units ordered.

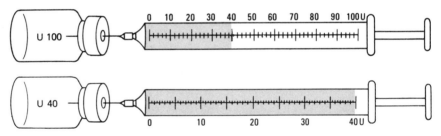

An accurate 40 U dose of two different concentrations of insulin

Both of the syringes in the above figure represent an accurate 40-unit dose of insulin. To assure accuracy you must remember (1) use the syringe calibrated for the concentration strength of insulin available, and (2) draw up an amount of units equal to the prescribed dose. Pay particular attention to the U 100 example, for that is the one you will use most frequently.

One last item that you must know about is that two insulins may be ordered to be administered at the same time (as is shown in the following figure). Most frequently it is a short- and an intermediate- or long-acting insulin that are ordered in combination. In most instances it is safe to prepare and administer them together. (Be sure to verify this.) After safety has been assured, you may measure these using the same syringe.

Be sure, however, that the same strength solutions of insulin are always used and that they correspond to the syringe you have chosen.

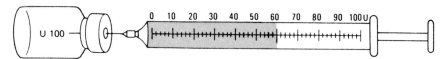

The prescribed dose is 10 units of a specific short-acting insulin and 50 units of long-acting insulin; the total dose is 60 units of insulin. Both short- and long-acting insulins are U 100 concentration.

▶   When you feel confident about these data, proceed to Activity Sheet 2.

Activity Sheet 2

1. Commonly used insulin is labeled U 100. What does this mean?

2. When preparing an insulin dosage, what fact must you take into account as you choose an insulin syringe?

For problems 3 through 12 indicate the amount of insulin that you would prepare by placing an arrow pointing to the proper calibration line on the syringe provided.

3. Insulin order: 68 U.

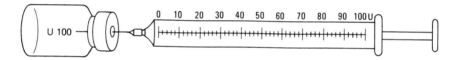

4. Insulin order: 20 U.

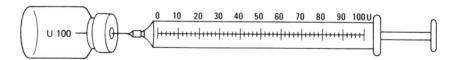

5. Insulin order: 44 U.

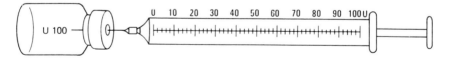

6. Insulin order: 40 U.

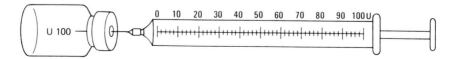

7. Insulin order: 10 U of short-acting insulin plus 52 U of long-acting insulin. At the completion of the preparation you should have drawn up a total of

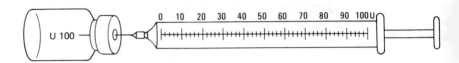

8. Insulin order: 12 U of short-acting insulin plus 46 U of long-acting insulin. At the completion of the preparation you should have drawn up a total of

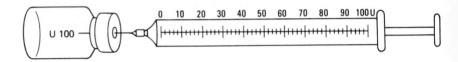

9. Insulin order: 10 U of short acting insulin plus 42 U of long acting insulin. At the completion of the preparation you should have drawn up a total of

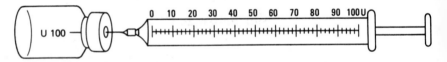

10. Insulin order: 75 U (U 100 insulin).

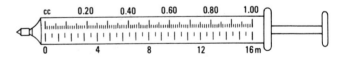

11. Insulin order: 44 U (U 100 insulin).

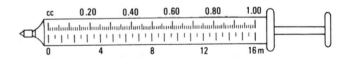

12. Insulin order: 82 U (U 100 insulin).

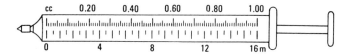

▶   Compare your answers with those at the end of this chapter. If you have mastered these questions, go to the text that follows. Otherwise review the previous text, correct your mistakes, and then go to the next section of text.

ADMINISTRATION OF U 500 INSULIN

Upon rare occasions U 500 insulin is required for patients. This is an extremely concentrated solution. It is 500 units of insulin per cubic centimeter. There does not exist, at present, a special U 500 insulin syringe for its administration. The manufacturer of the drug recommends the use of a tuberculin syringe to measure a prescribed dose. Therefore, to calculate a prescribed dose use the same process discussed in the previous section of this chapter when a tuberculin syringe was used to administer U 100 insulin.

Example

Administer 125 U of U 500 insulin.

Proportion Equation of Two Ratios

Dosage on hand   Dosage desired

$$\frac{500\ U}{1\ cc} = \frac{125\ U}{x\ cc}$$

$$500x = 125$$

$$x = \frac{125}{500} = \frac{1}{4} \text{ or } 0.25 \text{ cc}$$

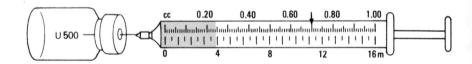

If a tuberculin syringe is not available, the U 100 insulin syringe may also be adapted and used. There are two acceptable methods for calculating the amount of fluid volume to be measured in units on the U 100 insulin syringe in order to administer a prescribed dose of U 500 insulin.

Example

Administer 125 U of U 500 insulin.
There are two methods that can be used to solve this problem:

Method 1
Because U 500 insulin is 5 times as concentrated as U 100 insulin, the number of units to be drawn up using the U 100 syringe and to be ad-

ministered should be one fifth (1/5) the number of prescribed units of U 500 insulin.

$$\frac{125}{5} \text{ U} = 25 \text{ U}$$

Remember that although you are drawing up a volume amount of 25 U on this syringe, a medication amount of 125 U is being drawn up to administer.

Method 2
This method merely adapts the one we have been using

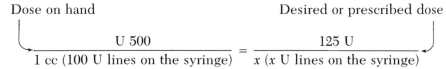

Dose on hand   Desired or prescribed dose

$$\frac{\text{U } 500}{1 \text{ cc (100 U lines on the syringe)}} = \frac{125 \text{ U}}{x \text{ (}x \text{ U lines on the syringe)}}$$

In this situation (U 500 insulin) the medication is available as 500 U/cc. The measuring instrument we have to measure this dose is a U 100 syringe. This is where the adaptation comes in. If we think of the U 100 on the syringe as representing that 1 cc, we can then use it in the above proportion; for if we draw up 100 U on the syringe we would have drawn up 500 U of insulin (known fact—500 U per 1 cc). With this in mind we can now calculate the dose:

$$\frac{500 \text{ U}}{1 \text{ cc (100 U)}} = \frac{125 \text{ U}}{x}$$

$$500x = 125 \times 100$$

$$500x = 12,500$$

$$x = 12,500 \div 500$$

$$x = 25 \text{ U}$$

We have thus calculated the above prescribed dose of 125 units of the U 500 insulin by two methods and have arrived at the same amount of fluid volume—$\frac{1}{4}$ cc (25 U)—that the person is to receive. These two methods can serve to verify each other. Therefore whichever method that is used should lead to the correct answer.

▶   When you feel confident about this material, proceed to Activity Sheet 3.

Activity Sheet 3

For the following prescribed dosages of U 500 insulin, calculate the fluid volume you would prepare in a tuberculin syringe and also draw a syringe and indicate the amount on it:

1. 150 U.

2. 200 U.

3. 250 U.

4. 180 U.

5. 210 U.

For the following prescribed dosages of U 500 insulin calculate the number of units to prepare in a U 100 insulin syringe:

6. 150 U.

7. 200 U.

8. 300 U.

9. 250 U.

10. 180 U.

11. 240 U.

12. 325 U.

13. 210 U.

► Compare your answers with those listed at the end of this chapter. If you have mastered these questions, take the posttest at the end of the chapter. If you have not mastered them, review the previous text and then correct your mistakes.

Posttest

1. State two commonly used measurements for medication other than those weight measures used in the apothecary or metric system.

2. A medication comes as 10,000 U/cc and you must add 15,000 U to a 500-cc bottle of intravenous fluid. Draw an arrow in the figure below to indicate the fluid volume you will prepare in this syringe:

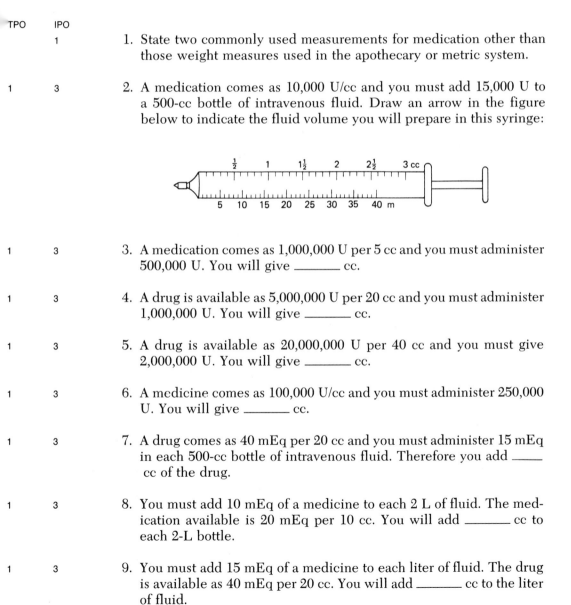

3. A medication comes as 1,000,000 U per 5 cc and you must administer 500,000 U. You will give _____ cc.

4. A drug is available as 5,000,000 U per 20 cc and you must administer 1,000,000 U. You will give _____ cc.

5. A drug is available as 20,000,000 U per 40 cc and you must give 2,000,000 U. You will give _____ cc.

6. A medicine comes as 100,000 U/cc and you must administer 250,000 U. You will give _____ cc.

7. A drug comes as 40 mEq per 20 cc and you must administer 15 mEq in each 500-cc bottle of intravenous fluid. Therefore you add _____ cc of the drug.

8. You must add 10 mEq of a medicine to each 2 L of fluid. The medication available is 20 mEq per 10 cc. You will add _____ cc to each 2-L bottle.

9. You must add 15 mEq of a medicine to each liter of fluid. The drug is available as 40 mEq per 20 cc. You will add _____ cc to the liter of fluid.

TPO	IPO	
1	3	10. You must administer three 20-mEq doses of a drug. It is available as 40 mEq per 30 cc. You will give _____ cc per dose and must be sure to have _____ cc of this medicine available.
1	3	11. You must give 30 mEq of a drug. It is available as 20 mEq per 15 cc. You will give _____ cc.
1	3	12. You must add 30 mEq of a drug to each 1000 cc of fluid. It is available as 2 mEq/cc. You will add _____ cc.
	4	13. Insulin is labeled U 100; what does this mean?
	5	14. When preparing an insulin dosage, what fact must you take into account as you choose an insulin syringe?
2		15. An insulin order is "6 U of clear insulin, 52 U of long-acting insulin." Draw an arrow indicating the calibration that is the total amount of insulin that should have been prepared.

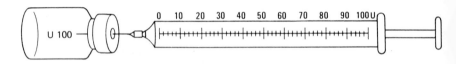

16. An insulin order is "5 U regular insulin, 35 U long-acting insulin." Draw an arrow indicating the calibration that is the total amount of insulin that should have been prepared.

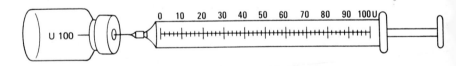

For the following two problems place an arrow indicating the accurate calibration line on the syringe that corresponds to the dose that you must administer:

17. Administer 275 U of U 500 insulin.

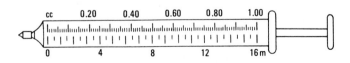

TPO   IPO

3   3   18. Administer 165 U of U 500 insulin.

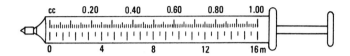

For the following prescribed dosages of U 500 insulin calculate the number of units to prepare in a U 100 syringe:

3   3   19. 400 U.

3   3   20. 350 U.

►   Compare your answers with those listed at the end of this chapter. If you have mastered this test, you are ready to start the next chapter. If you have not mastered this test, note the number next to the item(s) you answered incorrectly. This will tell you which objective you did not achieve. Return to the text and review. Then return to the activity sheets and practice appropriate items. Then recalculate the items you answered incorrectly on this test. After this take the pretest of this chapter as a second posttest. When you have corrected this test, you should be ready to proceed to the next chapter.

Answers for Chapter 5

PRETEST

1. Unit; milliequivalent	2. 3	3. 2.5
4. 2.5	5. 3	6. 0.5
7. 22.5	8. 4	9. 10
10. 30	11. 7.5	12. 20

13. There are 100 U of insulin per cc.
14. It must be calibrated according to the strength insulin you are using; for example, U 100 insulin, U 100 syringe.
15. 62 U

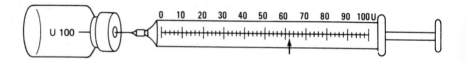

16. 40 U

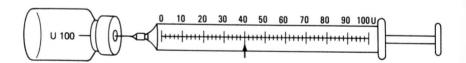

17.

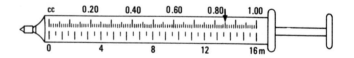

18.

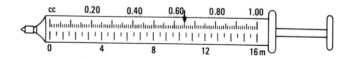

136

19. 75 U
20. 35 U

ACTIVITY SHEET 1

1. Units; milliequivalents
2. $1\frac{2}{3}$
3. 7.5
4.

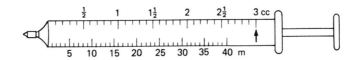

5. 3
6. 2
7. 15
8. 3
9. 22.5
10. 1.5
11. 3
12.

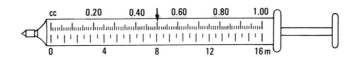

13. 2
14. 30
15. 6
16. 15
17. 90
18. 2.5
19. 15
20. 6 mEq; 3 cc

ACTIVITY SHEET 2

1. U 100: 100 units of insulin per cc.
2. It must correspond to the strength insulin being utilized; for U 100 insulin use a U 100 syringe.

3. 68 U

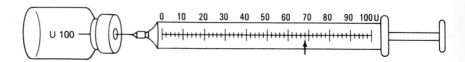

4. 20 U

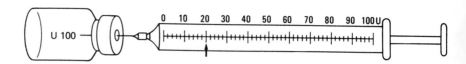

5. 44 U

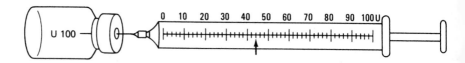

6. 40 U

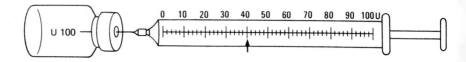

7. 62 U

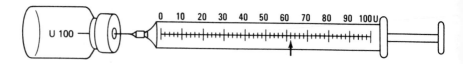

8. 58 U

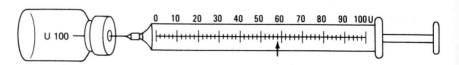

9. 52 U

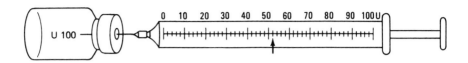

10. 75 U—0.75 cc

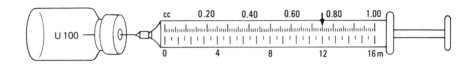

11. 44 U—0.44 cc

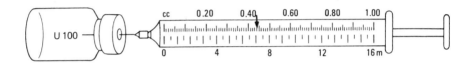

12. 82 U—0.82 cc

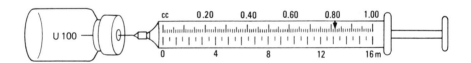

ACTIVITY SHEET 3

1. 0.3 cc

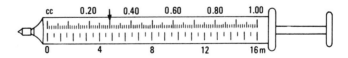

2. 0.4 cc

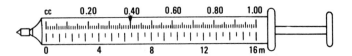

3. 0.5 cc

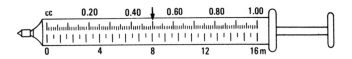

4. 0.36 cc

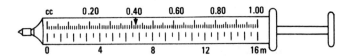

5. 0.42 cc

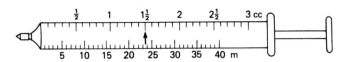

6. 30 U
7. 40 U
8. 60 U
9. 50 U
10. 36 U
11. 48 U
12. 65 U
13. 42 U

POSTTEST

1. Unit; milliequivalent
2.

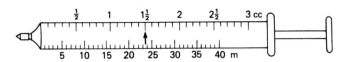

3. 2.5
4. 4
5. 4
6. 2.5
7. 7.5
8. 5
9. 7.5
10. 15, 45
11. 22.5
12. 15
13. There are 100 units of insulin per cc.
14. It must be calibrated according to the strength insulin you are using, for example, U 100 insulin, U 100 syringe.
15. 58 U

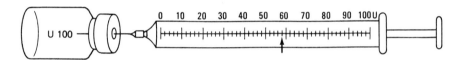

16. 40 U

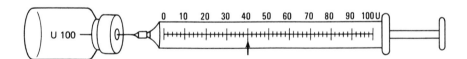

17. 0.55 cc

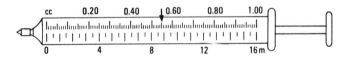

18. 0.33 cc

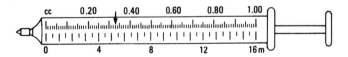

19. 80 U
20. 70 U

6 | *Household Measures*

TERMINAL PERFORMANCE OBJECTIVES

1. Given a volume in one household measure, the reader is able to convert it into another household measure.
2. Given a dosage contained in a household measure, the reader is able to calculate the amount of medication to be administered in that household measure for a prescribed dose.
3. Given a dosage contained in a household measure, the reader is able to calculate the amount of medication to be given in another household measure.

INTERMEDIATE PERFORMANCE OBJECTIVES

After studying the text, the reader is able to do the following:

1. List the five commonly used units of household measures used in drug administration.
2. Write the abbreviations used for the five household measures.
3. Write the meaning of a given abbreviation used in household measures.
4. List the four equivalents used in household measures.
5. Convert drops to teaspoonfuls.
6. Convert teaspoonfuls to drops.
7. Convert tablespoonfuls to teaspoonfuls.
8. Convert teaspoonfuls to tablespoonfuls.

9. Convert tablespoonfuls to ounces.
10. Convert ounces to tablespoonfuls.
11. Convert teaspoonfuls to ounces.
12. Convert ounces to teaspoonfuls.
13. Convert ounces to cups.
14. Convert cups to ounces.
15. Calculate the amount of teaspoonfuls, tablespoonfuls, or ounce to administer for a prescribed dose.
16. Calculate the amount of fluid volume to be administered for a prescribed dose when it is available diluted in another unit of fluid volume measure.

► If you feel confident that you can perform these behaviors, take the pretest. If you feel that you cannot perform these behaviors, begin this chapter by memorizing the data in the text.

Pretest

TPO	IPO	
	1	1. List five household measures used in the administration of drugs.
	2	2. Abbreviate: (a) teaspoon (b) tablespoon (c) cup (d) ounce (e) drop
	3	3. State the meaning of: (a) gtt (b) oz (c) T (d) c (e) t
	4.	4. Equivalents: (a) T = _____ t (b) 8 oz = _____ c (c) 2 T = _____ oz

TPO 1   IPO 5–14

5. Convert:
(a) 4 T   = _____ t   (b) 15 t   = _____ T
(c) 9 T   = _____ oz   (d) 5 oz   = _____ T
(e) 18 t   = _____ oz   (f) 6 oz   = _____ t
(g) 12 oz   = _____ c   (h) $1\frac{1}{4}$ c   = _____ oz

TPO 2   IPO 15

6. A drug comes as 125 mg/T and you must administer 0.25 g. You will give _____ T.

TPO 2   IPO 15

7. Give 0.25 mg. The medicine is available as 0.5 mg/t. Give _____ t.

TPO 2   IPO 12,15,16

8. A medicine comes as 375 mg/oz. You must give 125 mg. You will give _____ oz or _____ t.

TPO 3   IPO 7,15,16

9. A medicine comes as 0.75 g/T and you must administer 250 mg. You will give _____ t.

TPO 3   IPO 12,15,16

10. A drug comes as 42 mcg/oz. You must administer 7 mcg. You will give _____ t.

TPO	IPO
3	9,15,16

11. A drug comes 0.125 mg/T. You must give 0.25 mg. You will give _____ oz.

3	8,10,12, 15,16

12. A drug comes 0.6 mg/oz. You must give 300 mcg. You will give _____ t; _____ T.

3	8,15,16

13. A drug comes 0.05 mg/t. You must administer 0.15 mg. You will give _____ T.

▶ Compare your answers with those listed at the end of this chapter. If you have mastered this test, you may omit this chapter and start the next. If you have not mastered this test, begin this chapter by memorizing the data in the text.

GENERAL INFORMATION

Upon occasion you will use common household measurements in the administration of drugs. You will probably encounter this situation most frequently when you are teaching patients and their families how to measure preparations at home. You will find that most of these situations involve the measurement of liquids. The following text should provide sufficient background to enable you to feel confident in dealing with these household measurements.

CONVERTING LIQUID MEASURES

The following household measures are commonly used in calculating drug dosages:

Unit of Measure	Abbreviations[a]	Equivalents
Drop	gtt	75 gtt ↔ t[b]
Teaspoon	t, tsp	1 T ↔ 3 t
Tablespoon	T,Tbs,Tbsp	1 oz ↔ 2 T
Ounce	oz	1 c ↔ 8 oz
Cup	c,C	

[a] Sometimes you will find a period following an abbreviation.
[b] This equivalent is rarely used because drops vary in size and when drops are prescribed, the specific dropper accompanies the medication.

Example

$$6 \text{ oz} = \underline{\hspace{1.5cm}} \text{ t.}$$

Proportion Method

To set up the proportion, look to the equivalents shown in the table above for establishing the first relationship. If no equivalent exists between the two items you have been given—that is, ounces and teaspoons—look for an equivalent that may be an intermediate to find what 1 ounce is in teaspoons. Here we realize 2 T = 1 oz, and we know that 1 T = 3 t. Now we are able to start:

$$\frac{1 \text{ T}}{3 \text{ t}} = \frac{2 \text{ T (1 oz)}}{x \text{ t}}$$

$$x = 6 \text{ t}$$

Thus, there are 6 t in 1 oz. To determine how many teaspoons are in 6 oz, we set up the following proportion:

$$\frac{1 \text{ oz}}{6 \text{ t}} = \frac{6 \text{ oz}}{x \text{ t}}$$

$$x = 6 \times 6$$

$$x = 36 \text{ t}$$

Example

A medication comes as 6 mg in 1 t and you must administer 18 mg. Calculate the number of teaspoons you will need of this medication.

Dose on hand: 6 mg/t
Desired dose: 18 mg

Proportion Method

$$\frac{6 \text{ mg}}{1 \text{ t}} = \frac{18 \text{ mg}}{x \text{ t}}$$

$$6x = 18$$

$$x = 18 \div 6$$

$$x = 3 \text{ t} \, (= 1 \text{ T})$$

It is better to administer 1 T, especially to children, who might not take the three separate teaspoonfuls.

▶   When you are confident of this material, complete the Activity Sheet.

Activity Sheet

1. List the five household measures used in the administration of drugs.

2. Write the meaning of the following abbreviations:
   (a) gtt = _____   (b) t = _____   (c) oz = _____
   (d) tbsp = _____   (e) tsp = _____   (f) T = _____
   (g) c = _____   (h) tbs = _____

3. List the three equivalents of household measures commonly utilized in the administration of drugs.

4. Abbreviate (where there is more than one abbreviation, be sure to list all of them):
   (a) drop   (b) cup   (c) teaspoon
   (d) ounce   (e) tablespoon

5. (a) 8 oz = _____ c   (b) 1 t = _____ gtt
   (c) 2 T = _____ oz   (d) 3 t = _____ T

6. (a) 30 gtt = _____ t   (b) 150 gtt = _____ t

7. (a) 3 t = _____ gtt   (b) 5 t = _____ gtt

8. (a) 4 T = _____ t   (b) 5 T = _____ t

9. (a) 1 t = _____ T   (b) 5 t = _____ T

10. (a) 4 T = _____ oz   (b) 7 T = _____ oz

11. (a) 6 oz = _____ T   (b) $4\frac{1}{2}$ oz = _____ T

12. (a) 6 oz = _____ c   (b) 2 oz = _____ c

13. (a) 12 t = _____ oz   (b) 15 t = _____ oz

14. (a) 3 oz = _____ t   (b) 5 oz = _____ t

15. $\frac{1}{4}$ c = _____ oz = _____ T = _____ t

16. (a) $2\frac{2}{3}$ T = _____ t   (b) $1\frac{1}{3}$ T = _____ t

17. (a) 5 t = _____ T   (b) 7 t = _____ T

18. (a) 9 T = _____ oz   (b) 15 T = _____ oz

19. (a) $3\frac{1}{2}$ oz = _____ T   (b) $5\frac{1}{2}$ oz = _____ T

20. (a) 9 t = _____ oz   (b) 13 t = _____ oz

21. (a) $2\frac{1}{2}$ oz = _____ t   (b) 5 oz = _____ t

22. (a) 12 oz = _____ c   (b) 10 oz = _____ c

23. A drug is available as 1 g/t and the patient must take 500 mg He should take _____ t.

24. A drug comes as 9 g/T and you must administer 3 g. You will give _____ t.

25. A drug comes 60 mg/oz and you must administer 15 mg. You will give _____ T.

26. A drug is available as 42 mg/oz and 7 mg is ordered. You will give _____ t.

27. A drug comes as 3 mg/gtt and you must administer 135 mg. You will give _____ gtt, _____ t.

28. A drug comes as 5 mg/gtt and you must administer 300 mg. You will give _____ t.

29. A medication comes as 0.025 mg/t and you must give a patient 50 mcg. You will administer _____ t.

30. A drug comes 102 mg per 2 T and you must administer 17 mg. You will give _____ t.

31. A drug comes 0.25 g per 2 t and you must administer 1000 mg. You will give _____ T.

32. A drug comes 0.4 mg per 2 oz and you must administer 50 mcg. You will give _____ T.

33. A drug is available as 120 mg/oz and you must administer 20 mg. You will give _____ T, _____ t.

34. A medication comes as 180 mg/oz and you must administer 30 mg. You will give _____ t.

▶ Compare your answers with those listed at the end of this chapter. If you have mastered these problems, take the posttest. If you have not mastered these problems, review the text, redo the incorrect problems on the Activity Sheet, and then you should be ready for the posttest.

Posttest

TPO	IPO	
	1	1. List the five household measures used in the administration of drugs.

2. | IPO 2 | 2. Abbreviate:
(a) cup   (b) drop   (c) teaspoon
(d) ounce   (e) tablespoon |

TPO   **IPO**

1   1.   1. List the five household measures used in the administration of drugs.

      2.   2. Abbreviate:
               (a) cup   (b) drop   (c) teaspoon
               (d) ounce   (e) tablespoon

      3.   3. State the meaning for:
               (a) T   (b) c   (c) t
               (d) gtt   (e) oz

      4.   4. Equivalents:
               (a) 3 t = _____ T   (b) 1 c = _____ oz   (c) 1 oz = _____ T

1   5–14   5. Convert:
               (a) 2 T   = _____ t   (b) 21 t   = _____ T

               (c) 10 T   = _____ oz   (d) $4\frac{1}{2}$ oz = _____ T

               (e) 30 t   = _____ oz   (f) 3 oz   = _____ t

               (g) 20 oz = _____ c   (h) $\frac{1}{4}$ c   = _____ oz

2   15   6. A medication comes as 0.5 mg/T. You must administer 0.25 mg. You will give _____ T.

2   15   7. You must give 0.25 mg. The medication is available as 0.125 mg/t. You will give _____ t.

2   12,15,16   8. A medication comes as 0.375 mg/oz. You must administer 0.125 mg. You will give _____ oz, _____ t.

3   7,15,16   9. A drug comes as 1.5 g/T. You must administer 500 mg. You will give _____ t.

3   12,15,16   10. A drug comes as 30 mg/oz. You must administer 5 mg. You will give _____ t.

TPO	IPO	
3	9,15,16	11. A drug comes as 0.05 mg/T. You must administer 0.1 mg. You will give _____ oz.
3	8,10,12 15,16	12. A drug comes as 0.6 g/oz. You must administer 300 mg. You will give _____ t, _____ T.
3	8,15,16	13. A drug comes as 0.25 g/t. You must administer 750 mg. You will give _____ T.

► Compare your answers with those listed at the end of this chapter. If you have mastered these problems, you are ready to start the next chapter. If you have answered any of these questions incorrectly, note the numbers of the objectives next to your incorrect questions. Review the text related to these items. Redo some problems on the activity sheet that are similar to the ones you did incorrectly on this posttest, then redo the incorrect posttest items. After this you should be ready to take the pretest of this chapter as a second posttest. Correct it, review it, and then continue to the next chapter.

Answers for Chapter 6

PRETEST

1. Tablespoon, cup, ounce, drop, teaspoon
2. (a) t, tsp   (b) T, Tbs, Tbsp   (c) c, C   (d) oz (e) gtt
3. (a) Drop   (b) Ounce   (c) Tablespoon   (d) Cup
   (e) Teaspoon
4. (a) 3   (b) 1   (c) 1
5. (a) 12   (b) 5   (c) $4\frac{1}{2}$ (d) 10   (e) 3   (f) 36

   (g) $1\frac{1}{2}$ (h) 10

6. 2   7. $\frac{1}{2}$ 8. $\frac{1}{3}$, 2

9. 1   10. 1   11. 1
12. 3, 1   13. 1

ACTIVITY SHEET

1. Drop, teaspoon, tablespoon, ounce, cup
2. (a) Drop   (b) Teaspoon   (c) Ounce   (d) Tablespoon
   (e) Teaspoon (f) Tablespoon   (g) Cup   (h) Tablespoon
3. 1 T = 3 t
   1 oz = 2 T
   1 c = 8 oz
4. (a) gtt   (b) c, C   (c) t, tsp   (d) oz   (e) T, Tbs, Tbsp
5. (a) 1   (b) 75   (c) 1   (d) 1
6. (a) $\frac{2}{5}$ (b) 2   7. (a) 225   (b) 375

8. (a) 12   (b) 15   9. (a) $\frac{1}{3}$ (b) $1\frac{2}{3}$

10. (a) 2   (b) $3\frac{1}{2}$ 11. (a) 12   (b) 9

12. (a) $\frac{3}{4}$ (b) $\frac{1}{4}$ 13. (a) 2   (b) $2\frac{1}{2}$

14. (a) 18   (b) 30   15. 2, 4, 12

16. (a) 8   (b) 4   17. (a) $1\frac{2}{3}$ (b) $2\frac{1}{3}$

18. (a) $4\frac{1}{2}$ (b) $7\frac{1}{2}$ 19. (a) 7   (b) 11

20. (a) $1\frac{1}{2}$ (b) $2\frac{1}{6}$ 21. (a) 15   (b) 30

22. (a) $1\frac{1}{2}$ (b) $1\frac{1}{4}$

23. $\frac{1}{2}$ 24. 1   25. $\frac{1}{2}$

26. 1   27. 45, $\frac{3}{5}$ 28. $\frac{4}{5}$

29. 2   30. 1   31. $2\frac{2}{3}$

32. $\frac{1}{2}$ 33. $\frac{1}{3}$, 1   34. 1

POSTTEST

1. Tablespoon, cup, ounce, drop, teaspoon
2. (a) c, C   (b) gtt   (c) t, tsp   (d) oz   (e) T, Tbs, Tbsp
3. (a) Tablespoon   (b) Cup   (c) Teaspoon   (d) Drop   (e) Ounce
4. (a) 1   (b) 8   (c) 2
5. (a) 6   (b) 7   (c) 5   (d) 9   (e) 5   (f) 18   (g) $2\frac{1}{2}$ (h) 2

6. $\frac{1}{2}$ 7. 2   8. $\frac{1}{3}$, 2

9. 1   10. 1   11. 1

12. 3, 1   13. 1

7 | *Conversion Between Metric and Household Measures*

TERMINAL PERFORMANCE OBJECTIVES

1. Given the weight of a person (in either pounds or kilograms) and the amount of active ingredient a person is to receive per kilogram of body weight, the reader is able to compute the total amount of a drug a person is to receive.

2. Given a prescribed dosage and an available medication, both of which are measured in the metric system, the reader is able to calculate the measurement of liquid medication to be administered in household measures.

3. Given the amount of fluid a person ingests in household measures, the reader is able to compute the equivalent amount of cubic centimeters (or milliliters).

4. Given a prescribed metric or household liquid measure to administer and the available medication concentration, the reader is able to calculate the amount of active ingredient that is being administered.

5. Given a temperature reading measured on either the Fahrenheit or Celsius/centigrade scale, the reader is able to convert it to the other scale and determine if a medication or treatment should be given.

6. Given a linear measure of inches and feet, the reader is able to convert it to centimeters and millimeters and vice versa.

INTERMEDIATE PERFORMANCE OBJECTIVES

After studying the text, the reader is able to:

1. State the conversion factor between pounds and kilograms.
2. Convert pounds to kilograms and kilograms to pounds.
3. State the conversion factors between liquid metric and household measures.
4. Convert drops to cubic centimeters (or milliliters).
5. Convert cubic centimeters (or milliliters) to drops.
6. Convert teaspoonfuls to cubic centimeters (or milliliters).
7. Convert cubic centimeters (or milliliters) to teaspoonfuls.
8. Convert tablespoons to cubic centimeters (or milliliters).
9. Convert cubic centimeters (or milliliters) to tablespoons.
10. Convert ounces to cubic centimeters (or milliliters).
11. Convert cubic centimeters (or milliliters) to ounces.
12. Convert a Fahrenheit reading to the Celsius/centigrade equivalent.
13. Convert a Celsius/centigrade reading to the Fahrenheit equivalent.
14. Convert feet and inches to centimeters.
15. Convert centimeters to feet and inches.
16. Convert inches to millimeters.
17. Convert millimeters to inches.

► If you feel that you already possess these skills, take the pretest. Otherwise, study the material in this chapter.

Pretest

1. (a) A person's body weight of 88 lb = _____ kg.
   (b) If the prescribed dosage is 0.375 mg/kg of body weight, this person should receive _____ mg of medication.

2. (a) A person's body weight of 209 lb = _____ kg.
   (b) If the prescribed dose is 20 mcg/kg of body weight, this person should receive _____ mcg of medication.

3. (a) 15 gtt = _____ cc   (b) 2 cc = _____ gtt

For questions 4 and 5, how much liquid should be given in household measures?

4. Prescribed dose: 45 mcg
   Dosage available: 15 mcg per 15 cc

5. Prescribed dose: 0.125 mg
   Dosage available: 0.375 mg per 15 cc

For questions 6 and 7, what is the total fluid intake in cubic centimeters?

6. Lunch: 6 oz soup
           12 oz soda
           4 oz pudding

7. Breakfast: 5 oz cooked cereal
           3 oz juice
           8 oz milk

For questions 8 through 12, calculate the amount of active ingredient of medication the person is receiving.

8. Person receives: 1 T, 1 t
   Medication available: 30 mg per 5 cc

TPO	IPO	
4	6,7,10, 11	9. Person receives: 1 oz, 1 t Medication available: 30 mcg per 15 cc
4	8,9	10. Person receives: 30 cc Medication available: 50 mcg/T
4	6,7	11. Person receives: 15 cc Medication available: 0.125 mg/t
4	10,11	12. Person receives: 15 cc Medication available: 0.5 mg per 2 oz
5	12	13. 103° F = _____ °C
5	13	14. 38°C = _____ °F
5	13	15. You are to administer a medication if the temperature rises above 38.8°C. The patient's temperature is 102.5°F. Should the medication be given?
5	12	16. An order reads: administer a specific treatment if the temperature rises above 103.5°F. The patient's temperature is 39.5°C. Should the treatment be given?
6	14	17. 3 ft 2 in. = _____ cm
6	15	18. 149.86 cm = _____ ft _____ in.
6	16	19. 3.5 in. = _____ mm
6	17	20. 114.3 mm = _____ in.

► Compare your answers with those at the end of this chapter. If you have answered all questions correctly, you may omit this chapter. Otherwise, begin to study the material in this chapter.

CONVERTING LIQUID MEASURES

Unit of Measure	Abbreviation	Conversion Factor
Teaspoon	t	1 t ↔ 5 cc
Tablespoon	T	1 T ↔ 15 cc
Ounce	oz	1 oz ↔ 30 cc
Drop	gtt	15–16 gtt ↔ 1 cc[a]
Cubic centimeter	cc	30 cc ↔ 1 oz
Milliliter	mL	30 mL ↔ 1 oz

[a] This conversion factor is rarely used because drops vary in size. When medication is ordered in drops, there is usually a medicine dropper provided with the medication.

You must be able to convert liquid metric measures to household measures so that you can instruct patients how to measure their medications accurately at home. The figure below shows a measuring cup, graduated in both scales, that you may use.

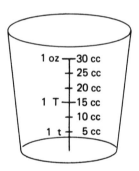

In converting these liquid factors to administer a prescribed dosage, remember that it is better to give whole measures than fractional amounts. For example, it is better to administer 2 t than $\frac{2}{3}$ T. It is also important to administer as few individual measures as is possible. Thus, 1 T is preferable to 3 t, even though both represent the same amount of fluid volume.

Another reason why you should be able to convert liquid measures is that fluid intake sheets are calculated in cubic centimeters (or milliliters) and frequently oral fluids are packaged measured in ounces.

Example

4 oz = _____ cc.

Use the conversion table to determine the relationship between the quantities being converted. Here you are dealing with oz and cc. The table indicates a relationship: 1 oz = 30 cc. To solve a conversion problem, this known relationship becomes the first ratio and will establish how you set up the quantities of the other ratio:

If you say $\dfrac{oz}{cc}$, then other side is also expressed as $\dfrac{oz}{cc}$.

If you say $\dfrac{cc}{oz}$, then other side is also expressed as $\dfrac{cc}{oz}$.

$$\begin{matrix} \text{Ratio of quantities} \\ \text{from conversion table} \end{matrix} = \begin{matrix} \text{Ratio of unknown} \\ \text{quantities} \end{matrix}$$

$$\dfrac{1 \text{ oz}}{30 \text{ cc}} = \dfrac{4 \text{ oz}}{x \text{ (cc)}}$$

$$x = 4 \times 30$$

$$x = 120 \text{ cc}$$

Example

45 cc = _____ T.

$$\begin{matrix} \text{Ratio of quantities} \\ \text{from conversion table} \end{matrix} = \begin{matrix} \text{Ratio of unknown} \\ \text{quantities} \end{matrix}$$

$$\dfrac{1 \text{ T}}{15 \text{ cc}} = \dfrac{x \text{ (T)}}{45 \text{ cc}}$$

$$15x = 45$$

$$x = 45 \div 15$$

$$x = 3 \text{ T}$$

Example

Desired dose: 0.5 g
Dosage available: 250 mg per 5 cc

The amount that should be given in household measures is _____ .

Computing Amount of Medication to Be Given

$$\frac{\text{Ratio of known facts}}{\text{(dose available)}} = \frac{\text{Ratio of unknown}}{\text{(desired dose)}}$$

$$\frac{250 \text{ mg}}{5 \text{ cc}} = \frac{500 \text{ mg } (0.5 \text{ g})}{x \text{ (cc)}}$$

$$250x = 5 \times 500$$

$$250x = 2500$$

$$x = 2500 \div 250$$

$$x = 10 \text{ cc}$$

Calculating the Amount to Be Given in Household Measures

$$\frac{\text{Ratio of quantities}}{\text{from conversion table}} = \frac{\text{Ratio of unknown}}{\text{(how much to give)}}$$

$$\frac{1 \text{ t}}{5 \text{ cc}} = \frac{x \text{ (t)}}{10 \text{ cc}}$$

$$5x = 10$$

$$x = 10 \div 5$$

$$x = 2 \text{ t}$$

► When you feel that you understand this material, complete Activity Sheet 1.

Activity Sheet 1

1. Equivalents:
   (a) _____ gtt ↔ 1 cc   (b) _____ t ↔ 5 cc
   (c) 1 T ↔ _____ cc   (d) 1 oz ↔ _____ cc

2. Convert:
   (a) 3 t   = _____ cc   (b) 30 gtt = _____ cc
   (c) 10 cc = _____ t   (d) 3 cc   = _____ gtt
   (e) 5 T   = _____ cc   (f) 225 cc = _____ T
   (g) 8 oz = _____ cc   (h) 135 cc = _____ oz
   (i) 5 t   = _____ cc   (j) 60 cc   = _____ t
   (k) 3 T   = _____ cc   (l) 60 cc   = _____ T
   (m) 3 oz = _____ cc   (n) 150 cc = _____ oz

For questions 3 through 12 calculate the amount that should be administered in household measures for the prescribed dosage.

3. Prescribed dose: 75 mcg
   Dosage available: 25 mcg per 10 cc

4. Prescribed dose: 150 mg
   Dosage available: 50 mg per 5 cc

5. Prescribed dose: 200 mg
   Dosage available: 50 mg per 5 cc

6. Prescribed dose: 360 mg
   Dosage available: 40 mg per 5 cc

7. Prescribed dose: 10 mg
   Dosage available: 30 mg per 15 cc

8. Prescribed dose: 15 mg
   Dosage available: 90 mg per 30 cc

9. Prescribed dose: 210 mg
   Dosage available: 30 mg per 5 cc

10. Prescribed dose: 250 mg
    Dosage available: 750 mg per 30 cc

11. Prescribed dose: 250 mg
    Dosage available: 0.5 g per 30 cc

12. Prescribed dose: 20 mg
    Dosage available: 15 mg per 15 cc

For questions 13 through 16 calculate the total fluid intake in cubic centimeters (or milliliters).

13. (a) Breakfast: 4 oz juice
        4 oz cooked
        cereal
        8 oz milk

    (b) Breakfast: 5 oz juice
        8 oz milk
        6 oz coffee

14. (a) Lunch: 5 oz tea
        3 oz juice
        4 oz soup

    (b) Lunch: 6 oz soup
        4 oz jello
        12 oz soda

15. (a) Supper: 5 oz soup
        3 oz juice
        8 oz coffee
        4 oz jello

    (b) Supper: 10 oz milk
        6 oz ice cream

16. Breakfast: 11 oz
    Lunch: 12 oz
    Supper: 15 oz
    Medicine: 4 oz
    Fluids between meals: 7 oz

For questions 17 through 24 calculate the amount of active ingredient of the medication that the person is receiving for the amount of fluid volume administered.

17. Person receives: 1 oz 1 T
    Medication labeled: 45 mg per 5 cc

18. Person receives: 1 T
    Medication labeled: 50 mg per 5 cc

19. Person receives: 1 oz 1 t
    Medication labeled: 20 mcg per 5 cc

20. Person receives: 1 t
    Medication labeled: 80 mg per 20 cc

21. Person receives: 30 cc
    Medication labeled: 120 mcg/T

22. Person receives: 15 cc
    Medication labeled: 120 mg/t

23. Person receives: 10 cc
    Medication labeled: 300 mg/oz

24. Person receives: 45 cc
    Medication labeled: 60 mcg/oz

► Compare your answers with those given at the end of this chapter. If you have answered all questions correctly, continue to the following section. Otherwise, review the previous section and correct your mistakes before continuing.

CONVERTING MEASURES OF WEIGHT AND DETERMINING DOSAGES ACCORDING TO BODY WEIGHT

As you review the literature accompanying drug packages, you will find that dosages are often stated to be administered as a specific amount of drug per kilogram of body weight. You therefore must be able to convert body weight measured in pounds to kilograms. This is easily done, as shown by the following examples.

Unit of Measure	Abbreviation	Conversion Factor
Pound	lb	2.2 lb ↔ 1 kg
Kilogram	kg	

Example

150 lb = _____ kg.

Ratio–Proportion Method

Ratio of quantities = Ratio of the unknown
from conversion table

$$\frac{2.2 \text{ lb}}{1 \text{ kg}} = \frac{150 \text{ lb}}{x \text{ (kg)}}$$

$$2.2x = 150$$

$$x = 150 \div 2.2$$

$$x = 68.18 \text{ kg}$$

Formula Method

Weight in kilograms = Weight in pounds ÷ 2.2

$$= 150 \div 2.2$$

$$= 68.18$$

Example

Person's weight: 154 lb

Medication dosage: 5 mg/kg of body weight

Calculate the number of milligrams of medication this person should receive in order to fulfill the medication dosage required.

Converting Body Weight

$$\text{Body weight in kilograms} = \text{Body weight in pounds} \div 2.2$$
$$= 154 \div 2.2$$
$$= 70$$

Determining the Dosage

Dosage
= Body weight in kg × amount of medication per kg of body weight

= 70 × 5 mg/kg of body weight

= 350 mg

▶ When you feel confident that you understand this material, complete Activity Sheet 2.

Activity Sheet 2

1. What is the conversion factor between pounds and kilograms?

2. Write the abbreviation for the following:
   (a) pounds   (b) kilogram

3. (a) A person weighs 180.4 lb. What is this weight in kilograms?
   (b) If the prescribed dosage is 10 mg/kg of body weight, this person should receive _____ mg of medication.

4. (a) A person weighs 143 lb. Express this weight in kilograms.
   (b) If the prescription calls for 0.5 mcg/kg of body weight, this person should receive _____ mcg of medication.

5. (a) A person weighs 165 lb. Express this in kilograms.
   (b) If the prescribed dosage is 3.5 mg/kg of body weight, this person should receive _____ mg of medication.

6. (a) A person weighs 110 lb. What is this weight in kilograms?
   (b) If the prescribed dosage is 0.125 mcg/kg of body weight, this person should receive _____ mcg of the medication.

7. (a) A person weighs 121 lb. Express this in kilograms.
   (b) If the prescribed dosage is 20 mg/kg of body weight, this person should receive _____ g of medication.

▶ Compare your answers with those listed at the end of this chapter. If you have answered all questions correctly, continue to the following section. Otherwise, review the text and recalculate the questions you answered incorrectly before continuing.

CONVERTING MEASURES OF TEMPERATURE AND DETERMINING TREATMENT FOR ELEVATED TEMPERATURES

When a person's temperature is elevated you may have to either administer certain medications or perform certain treatments.

Although at one time temperatures were normally reported using the Fahrenheit scale, today the Celsius/centigrade scale is being used with increasing frequency. In most instances there will be a graph, chart, or some sort of guide available to assist you in converting between these two scales. If no such guide is available, however, you may use the following conversion formulas:

$$\boxed{\begin{array}{c} \textit{Fahrenheit to Celsius} \\[2mm] °C = \dfrac{5}{9}\,(°F - 32°) \end{array}}$$

Example

$98.6°F = \underline{\hspace{2cm}} °C.$

$°C = \dfrac{5}{9}(°F - 32)$

$= \dfrac{5}{9}(98.6 - 32)$ Remember to perform the operation within the parentheses before multiplying.

$°C = \dfrac{5}{9}(66.6) = \dfrac{333}{9}$

$°C = 37$

$$\begin{array}{|c|}
\hline
\textit{Celsius to Fahrenheit} \\[4pt]
°F = \dfrac{9}{5}°C + 32 \\
\hline
\end{array}$$

Example

$$37°C = \underline{\qquad} °F.$$

$$°F = \frac{9}{5}°C + 32$$

$$= \frac{9}{5}(37) + 32 \qquad \text{Remember to multiply before performing addition.}$$

$$°F = 66.6 + 32$$

$$°F = 98.6$$

▶ When you feel confident that you understand this material, complete Activity Sheet 3.

Activity Sheet 3

1. 38.8°C = _____ °F   2. 103.6°F = _____ °C

3. 37.5°C = _____ °F   4. 105°F = _____ °C

5. The doctor orders an antipyretic drug if the patient's temperature reaches 38.5°C. It is currently 101.5°F. Would you give this drug?

6. The doctor wishes to be called if the patient's temperature is above 102°F. Will you call the doctor if patient's temperature is 39°C?

7. The patient is to be placed on a cooling mattress if his or her temperature exceeds 39.5°C. The patient's temperature is 103.3°F. What will you do?

8. The medication order reads:
   (a) For a temperature of 38°C and above take the patient's temperature every 2 hours.
   (b) For a temperature between 38.5° and 39.6°C administer a prescribed medication.
   (c) For a temperature of 39.8°C or above, contact the physician on call.
   The patient's temperature is 104°F. What should be done?

▶ Compare your answers with those listed at the end of this chapter. If you have answered all these questions correctly, continue to the next section. Otherwise, review the previous section and correct your mistakes before proceeding.

CONVERTING LINEAR MEASURE

In certain instances, you may need to convert linear measure. The following equivalents will help you with these conversions.

```
Abbreviations
  m = meter
 cm = centimeter
mm = millimeter
 ft = foot
 in. = inch
```

```
Equivalents
     1 ft = 12 in.
39.4 in. = 1 m = 100 cm
   1 in. = 2.54 cm = 25.4 mm
```

```
Symbols
   inch "
foot, feet '
```

Example

A child is 3 ft 4 in. tall. This is equal to _____ cm.

Formula Method
(a) *Change height to inches.*

$$\text{Height in inches} = \text{Height in feet} \times 12$$

$$= 3 \times 12$$

$$= 36$$

$$3 \text{ ft } 4 \text{ in.} = 36 \text{ in.} + 4 \text{ in.}$$

$$= 40 \text{ in.}$$

(b) *Convert in. to cm.*

$$\text{Height in cm} = \text{Height in inches} \times 2.54$$

$$= 40 \times 2.54$$

$$= 101.6$$

Ratio–Proportion Method

(a) *Change height to inches.*

Known ratio from
conversion table = Unknown ratio

$$\frac{12 \text{ in.}}{1 \text{ ft}} = \frac{x}{3 \text{ ft}}$$

$$x = 12 \times 3$$

$$x = 36 \text{ in.}$$

$$3 \text{ ft } 4 \text{ in.} = 36 \text{ in.} + 4 \text{ in.}$$

$$= 40 \text{ in.}$$

(b) *Convert in. to cm.*

$$\frac{1 \text{ in.}}{2.54 \text{ cm}} = \frac{40 \text{ in.}}{x}$$

$$x = 40 \times 2.54$$

$$x = 101.6$$

▶ When you feel confident that you understand this material, complete Activity Sheet 4.

Activity Sheet 4

1. 4 ft 3 in. = _____ in. = _____ cm

2. 5 ft 2 in. = _____ in. = _____ cm

3. 2 ft 11 in. = _____ in. = _____ cm

4. 139.7 cm = _____ in. = _____ ft _____ in.

5. 167.64 cm = _____ in. = _____ ft _____ in.

6. 2.5 in. = _____ mm

7. 3 in. = _____ mm

8. 60 mm = _____ in.

9. 90 mm = _____ in.

10. 50 in. = _____ cm = _____ mm

► Compare your answers with those at the end of this chapter. If you have answered all questions correctly, take the posttest. Otherwise, review the text of the previous section and correct your mistakes before taking the posttest.

Posttest

TPO	IPO
1	2

1. (a) A person weighs 187 lb. Express this in kilograms.
   (b) If the prescribed dosage is 2.2 mg/kg of body weight, this person should receive _____ mg of medication.

TPO	IPO
1	2

2. (a) A person weighs 99 lb. Express this in kilograms.
   (b) If the prescribed dosage is 100 mcg/kg of body weight, this person should receive _____ mg of medication.

IPO
4,5

3. (a) 15 gtt = _____ cc   (b) 7 cc = _____ gtt

For questions 4 and 5 calculate the amount of fluid a person should receive in household measures to administer the prescribed dosage.

TPO	IPO
2	6,7

4. Prescribed dose: 65 mcg
   Medication label: 130 mcg per 10 cc

TPO	IPO
2	8,11

5. Prescribed dose: 750 mg
   Medication label: 250 mg per 15 cc

For questions 6 and 7 calculate the fluid intake in cubic centimeters.

TPO	IPO
3	11

6. Lunch: 9 oz milkshake
          5 oz soup
          3 oz jello

TPO	IPO
3	11

7. Breakfast: 6 oz juice
              4 oz cooked cereal
              8 oz milk

For questions 8 through 11 calculate the amount of active ingredient that the person is receiving.

TPO	IPO
4	6–9

8. Person receives: 1 T 1 t
   Medication label: 15 mcg per 5 cc

176

TPO	IPO	
4	6,7 10,11	9. Person receives: 1 oz 1 t Medication label: 5 mg per 5 cc
4	10,11	10. Prescribed dose: 15 cc Medication label: 0.25 mcg/oz
4	6,7	11. Person receives: 15 cc Medication label: 0.125 mg/t
4	6,7 10,11	12. Person receives: 1 t Medication labeled: 72 mg per 30 cc
5	12	13. 101°F = _____ °C
5	13	14. 37.8°C = _____ °F
5	13	15. You are to administer a medication if the patient's temperature rises above 39.2°C. The patient's temperature is 101.5°F. Should the medication be given?
5	14	16. An order reads for a specific medication to be administered if the patient's temperature rises above 103.5°F. The patient's temperature is 39.8°C. Should the medication be given?
6	14	17. 4 ft 5 in. = _____ cm
6	15	18. 99.06 cm = _____ ft _____ in.
6	16	19. 5 in. = _____ mm
6	17	20. 254 mm = _____ in.

▶   Compare your answers with those listed at the end of this chapter. If you have answered all questions correctly, move on to the next chapter. Otherwise, note the number next to each test item you answered incorrectly, return to the appropriate text, review it, and practice appropriate items on the activity sheets. After you have corrected your mistakes on the posttest, take the pretest of this chapter as a second posttest. Once you have mastered the second posttest, you are ready to begin the next chapter.

Answers for Chapter 7

PRETEST

1. (a) 40   (b) 15   2. (a) 95   (b) 1900
3. (a) 1 cc   (b) 30 to 32   4. 1 oz 1 T
5. 1 t   6. 660
7. 480   8. 120 mg
9. 70 mcg   10. 100 mcg
11. 0.375 mg   12. 0.125 mg
13. 39.4   14. 100.4
15. Yes   16. No
17. 96.52   18. 4 ft 11 in.
19. 88.9   20. 4.5

ACTIVITY SHEET 1

1. (a) 15 to 16   (b) 1   (c) 15   (d) 30
2. (a) 15   (b) 2   (c) 2   (d) 45 to 48   (e) 75   (f) 15
   (g) 240   (h) $4\frac{1}{2}$ (i) 25   (j) 12   (k) 45   (l) 4
   (m) 90   (n) 5
3. 1 oz   4. 1 T
5. 1 T 1 t   6. 1 oz 1 T
7. 1 t   8. 1 t
9. 1 oz 1 t   10. 2 t
11. 1 T   12. 1 T 1 t
13. (a) 480   (b) 570   14. (a) 360   (b) 660
15. (a) 600   (b) 480   16. 1470
17. 405 mg   18. 150 mg
19. 140 mcg   20. 20 mg
21. 240 mcg   22. 360 mg
23. 100 mg   24. 90 mcg

ACTIVITY SHEET 2

1. 2.2 lb ↔ 1 kg
2. (a) lb (b) kg
3. (a) 82 (b) 820
4. (a) 65 (b) 32.5
5. (a) 75 (b) 262.5
6. (a) 50 (b) 6.25
7. (a) 55 (b) 1.1

ACTIVITY SHEET 3

1. 101.8
2. 39.77 ≈ 39.8
3. 99.5
4. 40.55 ≈ 40.6
5. Yes
6. Yes
7. Place them on the mattress.
8. Selection (c) and also (a)

ACTIVITY SHEET 4

1. 51, 129.54
2. 62, 157.48
3. 35, 88.9
4. 55, 4, 7
5. 66, 5, 6
6. 63.5
7. 76.2
8. 2.36
9. 3.54
10. 127, 1270

POSTTEST

1. (a) 85 (b) 187
2. (a) 45 (b) 4.5
3. (a) 1 cc (b) 105 to 112
4. 1 t
5. 1 oz 1 T
6. 510
7. 540
8. 60 mcg
9. 35 mg
10. 0.125 mcg
11. 0.375 mg
12. 12 mg
13. 38.3
14. 100
15. No
16. Yes
17. 134.62
18. 3 ft 3 in.
19. 127
20. 10

8 | *Intravenous Flow Rates*

TERMINAL PERFORMANCE OBJECTIVES

1. Given a prescribed volume of solution to administer intravenously over a specified time span, the reader is able to calculate the flow rate (number of drops per minute) at which to set the infusion or transfusion.
2. Given the flow rate at which a solution is being administered intravenously, the reader is able to calculate the amount of fluid volume a person is receiving within a specified time interval.

INTERMEDIATE PERFORMANCE OBJECTIVES

After studying the text, the reader is able to:

1. State one's mathematical responsibilities in regard to the intravenous administration of fluid.
2. Explain why flow rates may vary but still deliver the same amount of fluid in a specified time period.
3. Explain why flow rates may be identical but deliver a different amount of fluid in a specified time period.
4. List the four most common drop equivalencies or drop factors for fluid administration sets currently in use.
5. Explain why one must check the literature that is enclosed in the fluid administration set before calculating the flow rate.

6. Calculate the number of cubic centimeters of fluid per hour a person is to receive, after being given the total fluid volume and the number of hours over which to administer the fluid.

7. Calculate the number of cubic centimeters of fluid per minute a person is to receive, after being given the number of cubic centimeters per hour that person is receiving.

8. Calculate the number of drops per minute that will deliver a specified fluid volume per minute, hour, and multiple hours.

9. Use the long or short method in the calculation of intravenous flow rates and fluid volume amounts.

10. Use a formula in the calculation of intravenous flow rates and fluid volume amounts.

11. Calculate the total fluid volume a person will receive, after being given the number of cubic centimeters of fluid per hour the person is receiving and the number of hours over which the fluid will be administered.

12. Calculate the number of hours or the fraction of an hour that it will take a specified fluid volume to be administered, after being given either the number of cubic centimeters per hour or the flow rate at which the fluid is being administered.

13. Calculate the number of cubic centimeters of fluid per hour a person is to receive, after being given the number of cubic centimeters per minute that person is receiving.

14. Calculate the amount of fluid volume a person is receiving per minute, hour, and in multiple hours, after being given the number of drops per minute an infusion is running.

▶ If you feel confident that you possess these skills, take the pretest that follows. Otherwise, begin to study the material in this chapter.

Pretest

TPO   IPO

1. What are your mathematical responsibilities in regard to the intravenous administration of fluids?

2. Why may flow rates vary but still deliver the same amount of fluid per hour?

3. Why may two intravenous flow rates be identical and yet deliver different amounts of fluid volume?

4. List four common IV administration set drop equivalencies or drop factors (that is, the number of drops that equal 1 cc).

5. Why must you check the literature that is enclosed in the fluid administration set before you calculate a flow rate?

6. A person is to receive 1200 cc (or mL) of fluid over 8 hours. How many cc/hr should this person receive?

7. If 3000 cc of fluid is to be absorbed over a 24-hour period, how many cc/hr should be administered?

8. The infusion rate is 120 cc/hr. How many cc/min is this?

9. The infusion rate is 10 cc/hr. How many cc/min is this?

For questions 10 through 14, calculate the flow rates for administration sets having the following equivalencies: (a) 15 gtt = 1 cc; (b) 12 gtt = 1 cc; (c) 10 gtt = 1 cc; and (d) 60 gtt = 1 cc.

10. The infusion rate is 2 cc/min. The flow rate should be
   (a)   (b)
   (c)   (d)

TPO	IPO
1	8

11. The infusion rate is ½ cc/min. The flow rate should be
(a)   (b)
(c)   (d)

| 1 | 8,9, or 10 |

12. The infusion rate is 180 cc/hr. The flow rate should be
(a)   (b)
(c)   (d)

| 1 | 8,9, or 10 |

13. The infusion rate is 125 cc/hr. The flow rate should be
(a)   (b)
(c)   (d)

| 1 | 8,9, or 10 |

14. If 1200 cc of fluid is to be absorbed over a 10-hour period, the flow rate should be
(a)   (b)
(c)   (d)

| 1 | 8,9, or 10 |

15. If 450 cc of blood is to be administered over a 3-hour period, the flow rate should be _____ .

| | 11 |

16. If a person receives 80 cc/hr, how much fluid will be received in 24 hours?

| | 11 |

17. If a person receives 125 cc/hr for the 8 hours you care for him or her, that person will receive _____ cc (or mL).

| | 12 |

18. If 2500 cc of fluid is ordered, and the patient is to receive 100 cc/hr, it will take _____ hours for the fluid to be administered.

| | 12 |

19. If 1500 cc of fluid is ordered, and the patient is to receive 75 cc/hr, it will take _____ hours for the fluid to be administered.

| 2 | 12 |

20. You find that there is 240 cc of fluid left. The flow rate is 30 gtt/min. The administration set equivalency is 15 gtt = 1 cc. How long will this fluid last?

| 2 | 12 |

21. You find that there is 60 cc of fluid left. The flow rate is 120 gtt/min. The administration set equivalency is 60 gtt = 1 cc. How long will this fluid last?

| 2 | 12 |

22. You find that there is 150 cc of fluid left. The flow rate is 30 gtt/min. The administration set equivalency is 10 gtt = 1 cc. How long will this fluid last?

TPO	IPO	
	13	23. An infusion instills 1.5 cc/min. How many cc/hr will be administered at this rate?
2	14	24. An intravenous flow rate is 40 gtt/min. The administration set equivalency is 10 gtt = 1 cc. Calculate the amount of fluid volume in cubic centimeters that this person is receiving (a) per minute, (b) per hour, and (c) during the 8 hours you are caring for him or her.
2	14	25. An intravenous flow rate is 45 gtt/min. The administration set equivalency is 60 gtt = 1 cc. Calculate the amount of fluid volume in cubic centimeters that this person is receiving (a) per minute, (b) per hour, and (c) during a 12-hour time period.

► Compare your answers with those at the end of this chapter. If you have answered all questions correctly, begin the next chapter. Otherwise, begin this chapter by reading the next section of text.

GENERAL INFORMATION

When intravenous fluids are ordered for patients, the physician prescribes the amount and various types of solutions to be administered as
well as the number of hours over which these fluids are to be infused.
For example, a nurse might receive the following order:

1. 1000 cc D5W

2. 1000 cc D5NS

3. 1000 cc D5 $\frac{1}{2}$ NS

Run these fluids over 24 hours.

The nurse then has the responsibility to calculate the number of cubic
centimeters per hour the patient must receive and the number of drops
per minute (the flow rate) at which to regulate the infusion.

The physician may also prescribe the type of fluid to be administered
and the number of cubic centimeters per hour a person is to receive. A
typical order would read NS @ 100 cc/hr. The nurse then need only
compute the flow rate at which to set the infusion.

In the process of calculating the flow rate, one of the most important
factors is the drop size. Drop size varies with the specific administration
set used. (See the figure below.) The size of the drop delivered by the
apparatus determines how many of those drops will equal 1 cc. (The
smaller the drop size the greater the number of drops needed to equal
1 cc of fluid volume.)

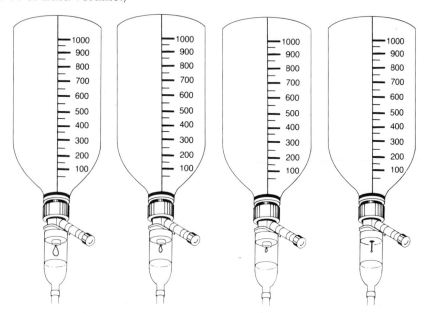

These four bottles with IV tubing illustrate drip chambers with drops of various sizes.

This explains why two intravenouses may be administered at different flow rates and yet deliver the same amount of fluid (the one with the slower flow rate has a larger drop size) and why two intravenouses may be given at the same flow rate and yet deliver different amounts of fluid (their drop sizes are not equal).

The most common sets that you will be using have the following drop equivalencies:

1. 15 gtt = 1 cc ⎫
2. 12 gtt = 1 cc ⎬ called a macrodrip or macrodrop set
3. 10 gtt = 1 cc ⎭
4. 60 gtt = 1 cc

The 60 gtt = 1 cc set is called a microdrip, pedidrip, or minidrip set. It is used with both bottle and bagged fluid preparations and is particularly useful for the slow administration of fluids or medicines and when fluid intake must be kept at a minimum, but an intravenous line maintained.

The literature pertaining to the infusion administration set must always be read to verify the number of drops that equals 1 cc. In subsequent sections of this chapter the process for calculating intravenous flow rates is explained. It should, however, be emphasized that when medicated solutions are administered it is safer to use an infusion pump. This is discussed in a subsequent chapter.

▶   When you feel that you understand this material, complete Activity Sheet 1.

Activity Sheet 1

1. After the physician has written the intravenous order, what are your mathematical responsibilities in regard to the intravenous administration of fluids?

2. Define flow rate.

3. What is the most important factor for you to know in order to calculate a flow rate?

4. Why may flow rates differ but still deliver the same amount of fluid in a specified time period?

5. Why may flow rates be identical in number of drops per minute but deliver different amounts of fluid in a specified time period?

6. List the four most common drop equivalencies.

7. Before you use an administration set, why must you check the accompanying literature?

▶ Compare your answers with those at the end of this chapter. If you have answered all questions correctly, continue to the text that follows. Otherwise review the previous text and correct your mistakes before continuing.

CALCULATING THE FLOW RATE—REGULAR THREE-STEP METHOD

There are a number of methods for calculating the flow rate for an intravenous infusion. This chapter explains how to use a number of different methods, and gives you practice with each of them, because individuals vary in the manner in which they learn and in what they find easy. It is suggested that you try each of the methods and then decide which you find easiest to remember and use.

Although the first method may initially appear somewhat long, it consists of a series of sequential steps. Once you become familiar with them, they will seem very logical and, therefore, easy to remember.

Example

Refer to the sample order in the previous section in which the nurse is asked to administer a total volume of 3000 cc over a 24-hour period. The fluid administration set was 15 gtt = 1 cc.

Three-Step Method

1. Calculate the number of **cubic centimeters per hour** the patient is to receive.

> Number of cc/hr =
> Total fluid volume ÷ number of hours fluid is to be administered

$$cc/hr = 3000 \ cc \div 24 \ hr$$

$$= 125$$

2. Calculate the number of **cubic centimeters per minute** the patient is to receive.

> Number of cc/min =
> Number of cc/hr ÷ 60 min (number of minutes in 1 hour)

$$cc/min = 125 \ cc/hr \div 60 \ min$$

$$= 2\frac{1}{12}$$

3. Calculate the **flow rate** (number of drops per minute) at which to set the intravenous flow.

Flow rate (gtt/min) =
 Number of cc/min × number of gtt/cc in particular set used

$$15 \text{ gtt} = 1 \text{ cc}$$
$$12 \text{ gtt} = 1 \text{ cc}$$
$$10 \text{ gtt} = 1 \text{ cc}$$

or

$$60 \text{ gtt} = 1 \text{ cc}$$

$$\text{Flow rate (gtt/min)} = 2\frac{1}{12} \text{ cc/min} \times 15 \text{ gtt/cc}$$

$$= \frac{25}{12} \times 15$$

$$= 31.25 \text{ or } 31\frac{1}{4} \approx 31$$

The final answer to this problem is to set the flow rate at 31 gtt/min to deliver 125 cc/hr and 3000 cc over a 24-hour period.

▶ When you feel that you understand this material, complete Activity Sheet 2.

Activity Sheet 2

For questions 1 through 5 calculate the number of cc/hr a person will receive for the given information.

1. A person is to receive 1800 cc over 24 hours.

2. A person is to receive 1500 cc over 12 hours.

3. A person is to receive 1000 cc over 24 hours.

4. A person is to receive 800 cc over 8 hours.

5. A person is to receive 600 cc over 12 hours.

For questions 6 through 10, calculate the number of cc/min a person will receive.

6. The infusion rate is 75 cc/hr.

7. The infusion rate is 125 cc/hr.

8. The infusion rate is 15 cc/hr.

9. The infusion rate is 100 cc/hr.

10. The infusion rate is 50 cc/hr.

For questions 11 through 27, calculate the flow rates for administration sets having the following equivalencies: (a) 15 gtt = 1 cc, (b) 12 gtt = 1 cc, (c) 10 gtt = 1 cc, and (d) 60 gtt = 1 cc.

11. The infusion rate is $1\frac{1}{4}$ cc/min. The flow rates should be

    (a)   (b)
    (c)   (d)

12. The infusion rate is $2\frac{1}{12}$ cc/min. The flow rates should be

(a)   (b)
(c)   (d)

13. The infusion rate is $\frac{25}{36}$ cc/min. The flow rates should be

(a)   (b)
(c)   (d)

14. The infusion rate is $1\frac{2}{3}$ cc/min. The flow rates should be

(a)   (b)
(c)   (d)

15. The infusion rate is $\frac{5}{6}$ cc/min. The flow rates should be

(a)   (b)
(c)   (d)

16. The infusion rate is 240 cc/hr. The flow rates should be
(a)   (b)
(c)   (d)

17. The infusion rate is 90 cc/hr. The flow rates should be
(a)   (b)
(c)   (d)

18. The infusion rate is 60 cc/hr. The flow rates should be
(a)   (b)
(c)   (d)

19. The infusion rate is 100 cc/hr. The flow rates should be
(a)   (b)
(c)   (d)

20. The infusion rate is 120 cc/hr. The flow rates should be
(a)   (b)
(c)   (d)

21. If 2000 cc of fluid is to be administered over a 10-hour period, the flow rates should be
(a)   (b)
(c)   (d)

22. If 1000 cc of fluid is to be administered over an 8-hour period, the flow rates should be
(a)   (b)
(c)   (d)

23. If 2400 cc of fluid is to be administered over a 24-hour period, the flow rates should be
(a)   (b)
(c)   (d)

24. If 2000 cc of fluid is to be administered over 16 hours, the flow rates should be
(a)   (b)
(c)   (d)

25. If 2000 cc of fluid is to be administered over 30 hours, the flow rates should be
(a)   (b)
(c)   (d)

26. If 1000 cc of fluid is to be administered over a 16-hour period, the flow rates should be
(a)   (b)
(c)   (d)

27. A person is to receive 1000 cc over a 4-hour period. The flow rates should be
(a)   (b)
(c)   (d)

For questions 28 through 30 calculate the flow rates for only the administration set 10 gtt = 1 cc, because blood is administered most frequently using this set.

28. A person is to receive 300 cc of blood over a 3-hour period.

29. A person is to receive 450 cc of blood in 2 hours.

30. A person is to receive 480 cc of blood over 4 hours.

▶ Compare your answers with those at the end of this chapter. If you have answered all questions correctly, continue to the text that follows. Otherwise, review the previous text and correct your mistakes before proceeding.

CALCULATING THE FLOW RATE—FORMULA METHOD

Some people prefer to use formulas to solve problems. Now that you have learned the three-step method for calculating the flow rate of an intravenous solution, we can introduce a formula that will allow you to solve a flow-rate problem in what appears to be one step. In order to illustrate that you will obtain the same answer whether you use the three-step method or the formula method, we shall solve the problem used previously to demonstrate the three-step method.

Example

Administer 3000 cc of fluid over a 24-hour period. The fluid administration set used is 15 gtt = 1 cc.

Formula Method

$$\text{Flow rate} = \frac{\text{Fluid volume} \times \text{number of gtt/cc (for the set being used)}}{\text{Time in minutes}}$$

$$= \frac{3000\ \text{cc} \times 15\ \text{gtt/cc}}{24\ \text{hr} \times 60\ \text{min/hr}} = \frac{\overset{50}{\cancel{3000}} \times 15}{\underset{1}{24 \times \cancel{60}}}$$

$$= \frac{50}{24} \times \frac{15}{1} = \frac{50}{\underset{8}{\cancel{24}}} \times \frac{\overset{5}{\cancel{15}}}{1}$$

$$= \frac{50}{8} \times \frac{5}{1} = \frac{\overset{25}{\cancel{50}}}{\underset{4}{\cancel{8}}} \times \frac{5}{1}$$

$$= \frac{25}{4} \times \frac{5}{1} = \frac{125}{4} = 31.25 \approx 31\ \text{gtt/min}$$

Actually, the formula method contains the same steps as the three-step method, as is illustrated on the opposite page. The only difference is that instead of dividing the problem into three discrete steps, all the information is inserted into a single formula. We can see this if we examine the data in the previous problem:

Comparing Three-Step and Formula Methods

$$\text{Flow rate} = \frac{3000 \times 15}{24 \times 60}$$

Step 1. Determine the number of cc/hr the person is receiving (fluid volume ÷ number of hours).

Step 2. Determine the number of cc/min the person is to receive (cc/hr ÷ 60 min/hr).

Step 3. Determine the flow rate, that is, the number of gtt/min at which to set the intravenous (cc/min × number of gtt/cc for the set being used).

▶ When you feel that you understand this material, complete Activity Sheet 3.

Activity Sheet 3

For problems 1 through 8, calculate the flow rates for administration sets having the following equivalencies: (a) 15 gtt = 1 cc; (b) 12 gtt = 1 cc; (c) 10 gtt = 1 cc; and (d) 60 gtt = 1 cc.

1. If 1500 cc of fluid is to be administered over 24 hours, the flow rates should be
   (a)   (b)
   (c)   (d)

2. If 2000 cc of fluid is to be administered over 24 hours, the flow rates should be
   (a)   (b)
   (c)   (d)

3. If 1200 cc of fluid is to be administered over 8 hours, the flow rates should be
   (a)   (b)
   (c)   (d)

4. If 560 cc of fluid is to be administered over 8 hours, the flow rates should be
   (a)   (b)
   (c)   (d)

5. The infusion rate is 50 cc/hr. The flow rates should be
   (a)   (b)
   (c)   (d)

6. The infusion rate is 75 cc/hr. The flow rates should be
   (a)   (b)
   (c)   (d)

7. The infusion rate is 85 cc/hr. The flow rates should be
   (a)   (b)
   (c)   (d)

8. The infusion rate is 40 cc/hr. The flow rates should be
   (a)   (b)
   (c)   (d)

For questions 9 through 12 calculate the flow rates for only the administration set 10 gtt = 1 cc, because blood is administered via this type set.

9. A person is to receive 225 cc of blood over 2 hours.

10. A person is to receive 480 cc of blood over 6 hours.

11. A person is to receive 450 cc of blood over 4 hours.

12. A person is to receive 500 cc of blood over 4 hours.

At times, you will have to administer what is called a fluid challenge. This involves giving a specified amount of fluid in a short period of time. For questions 13 through 15, calculate the flow rate assuming that the administration set used is 15 gtt = 1 cc. Utilization of this method to calculate the rate of flow for the solution is safe, quick, and easy.

13. Administer 250 cc of D5 $\frac{1}{2}$ NS in 20 minutes.

14. Administer 250 cc of D5 $\frac{1}{4}$ NS in 45 minutes.

15. Administer 200 cc of D5 $\frac{1}{2}$ NS in 30 minutes.

▶ Compare your answers with those at the end of this chapter. If you have answered all questions correctly, continue to the text that follows. Otherwise, review the previous text and correct your mistakes before proceeding.

CALCULATING THE FLOW RATE—SHORTENED METHOD

The third method that can be used to calculate intravenous flow rates is short and easy to master. In the previous section a formula was developed from the three-step method for calculating intravenous flow rates: in the shortened method, we need only know the cc/hr a person is to receive and divide that number by a certain "special number":

Flow rate = cc/hr ÷ "special number"

This method is very practical in clinical practice. In the course of the day a patient's intravenous rate is very frequently changed and the fluid and administration set remains the same. This being so, to determine the new flow rate is relatively easy. It merely entails dividing the new intravenous rate (cc/hr) by the special number for the administration set being used.

The special number will vary depending upon the administration set used. You will become very familiar with the ones used in your setting because you will be dealing with them every day. The following are the special numbers you should memorize to prepare yourself for most situations:

Administration Set	Special Number
15 gtt = 1 cc	4
12 gtt = 1 cc	5
10 gtt = 1 cc	6
60 gtt = 1 cc	1

Example

An intravenous has been ordered to run at 100 cc/hr and you have set the flow rate at 20 gtt/min. The administration set is 12 gtt = 1 cc. New orders have been written and now the person is to receive 80 cc/hr. What should you now set the flow rate at?

To Solve

Flow rate = cc/hr ÷ special number

= 80 ÷ 5

= <u>16</u> gtt/min

Example

A person is to receive 3000 cc of fluid over 24 hours. The administration set is 15 gtt = 1 cc. (This is the same problem used to illustrate the other two methods. Once again we will obtain the same answer.)

To Solve
In the previous example we knew the number of cc/hr. Here we must first find this number:

$$\text{Number of cc/hr} = \text{fluid volume} \div \text{number of hours}$$

$$= 3000 \div 24$$

$$= 125$$

Now we insert this number into the shortened method:

$$\text{Flow rate} = \text{cc/hr} \div \text{special number}$$

$$= 125 \div 4$$

$$= 31.25 \approx 31 \text{ gtt/min}$$

Rationale for the Shortened Method

You **need not memorize** this section but you should read it in order to understand how this shortened method was developed. It will probably be easier to understand if you reread the three-step method in the first section of this chapter before you read the text that follows.

Guide for a Set in Which 15 gtt = 1 cc

$$\boxed{\text{Flow rate} = \text{cc/hr} \div 4}$$

Rationale
In the three-step method you divided the cc/hr by 60 (to obtain the cc/min) and multiplied this by 15 (the number of gtt in 1 cc) to obtain the flow rate, that is,

$$\frac{1}{60} \times 15 = \frac{1}{4}$$

This 1/4 is the same as dividing the number of cc/hr by the special number 4.

Guide for a Set in Which 12 gtt = 1 cc

$$\boxed{\text{Flow rate} = \text{cc/hr} \div 5}$$

Rationale

In the long method you divided the number of cc/hr by 60 and then multiplied by 12, that is,

$$\frac{1}{60} \times 12 = \frac{12}{60} = \frac{1}{5}.$$

This 1/5 is the same as dividing the number by the special number 5.

Guide for a Set in Which 10 gtt = 1 cc

$$\boxed{\text{Flow rate} = \text{cc/hr} \div 6}$$

Rationale

In the long method you divided the number of cc/hr by 60 and then multiplied by 10 to obtain the flow rate, that is,

$$\frac{1}{60} \times 10 = \frac{10}{60} = \frac{1}{6}$$

This 1/6 is the same as dividing the number of cc/hr by the special number 6.

Guide for Microdrip Chambers—60 gtt = 1 cc

$$\boxed{\text{Flow rate} = \text{cc/hr} \div 1}$$

Use the fact that the number of cc/hr indicates the flow rate (number of gtt/min) at which to regulate the microdrip. That is, for 90 cc/hr set the rate at 90 microgtt/min; for 40 cc/hr set the rate at 40 microgtt/min.

Rationale

In the long method you divided the number of cc/hr by 60 and then multiplied by 60 gtt/min, that is,

$$\frac{1}{60} \times 60 = 1$$

This 1 is the same as dividing by the special number 1, or using the same numerical value.

▶   When you feel that you understand this material, complete Activity Sheet 4.

Activity Sheet 4

1. With regard to the short method, indicate the special number that you would use to divide into the number of cc/hr to find the number of gtt/min at which to regulate the following sets:
   (a) 15 gtt = 1 cc   (b) 12 gtt = 1 cc
   (c) 10 gtt = 1 cc   (d) 60 gtt = 1 cc

2. Write out the guides for the short method utilized to calculate flow rates.
   (a)   (b)
   (c)   (d)

For questions 3 through 10, calculate the flow rates for administration sets having the following equivalents: (a) 15 gtt = 1 cc, (b) 12 gtt = 1 cc, (c) 10 gtt = 1 cc, and (d) 60 gtt = 1 cc.

3. A person is to receive 1200 cc over a 24-hour period. The flow rates should be
   (a)   (b)
   (c)   (d)

4. A person is to receive 900 cc over a 12-hour period. The flow rates should be
   (a)   (b)
   (c)   (d)

5. A person is to receive 600 cc over a 24-hour period. The flow rates should be
   (a)   (b)
   (c)   (d)

6. A person is to receive 960 cc over a 24-hour period. The flow rates should be
   (a)   (b)
   (c)   (d)

7. A person is to receive 60 cc/hr. The flow rates should be
   (a)   (b)
   (c)   (d)

8. A person is to receive 90 cc/hr. The flow rates should be
   (a)   (b)
   (c)   (d)

9. A person is to receive 144 cc/hr. The flow rates should be
   (a)   (b)
   (c)   (d)

10. A person is to receive 120 cc/hr. The flow rates should be
    (a)   (b)
    (c)   (d)

For the following two questions, calculate the flow rates for blood administered using a set having the equivalent 10 gtt = 1 cc.

11. Administer 360 cc of blood over a 4-hour period.

12. Administer 240 cc of blood over a 2-hour period.

With your previous experience you should now be able to formulate the short method for any fluid administration set, once you know the number of drops that equals 1 cc.

13. The set's equivalency is 20 gtt = 1 cc.
    (a) The special number would be _____ .
    (b) Problem: To administer 240 cc in 2 hours, the flow rate for this set should be _____ gtt/min.

14. The equivalent is 6 gtt = 1 cc.
    (a) The special number would be _____ .
    (b) Problem: To administer 300 cc over 2 hours, the flow rate for this set should be _____ gtt/min.

▶ Compare your answers with those listed at the end of this chapter. If you have answered all questions correctly, proceed on to the text that follows. Otherwise, review the previous text and correct your mistakes before proceeding.

CALCULATING THE FLUID VOLUME RECEIVED OVER A SPECIFIC TIME SPAN

Given the amount of fluid to be administered, you have thus far learned the basic mathematics necessary to calculate the appropriate flow rate. Sometimes you will need to work in the opposite direction, that is, you will know how much fluid a person is receiving per hour and will need to calculate how much fluid the patient receives during a specified time period.

> Fluid volume = Number of cc/hr × number of hr

Example

If a person is being given 125 cc/hr, how much fluid will be received in an 8-hour period?

To Solve

$$\text{Fluid volume} = 125 \text{ cc/hr} \times 8 \text{ hr}$$
$$= 1000 \text{ cc}$$

▶ When you feel that you understand this material, complete Activity Sheet 5.

Activity Sheet 5

Calculate the fluid volume (cc) received in the following situations:

1. A person receives 150 cc of fluid for 10 hours.

2. A person receives 110 cc of fluid for 24 hours.

3. A person receives 100 cc of fluid for 12 hours of the day and 75 cc of fluid for the remaining 12 hours.

4. A person is to receive 50 cc of fluid per hour for the 12 hours you are taking care of him or her.

5. A person is to receive 80 cc of fluid per hour for the 8 hours you care for him or her.

▶ Compare your answers with those at the end of this chapter. If you have answered all questions correctly, continue to the text that follows. Otherwise, review the previous text and correct your mistakes before proceeding.

CALCULATING THE INFUSION TIME FOR A SPECIFIC VOLUME

Suppose that a patient's intravenous is running at the specified flow rate. You know how much fluid remains in the bottle. You want to know how long it will last. To make this calculation, use one of the following formulas:

$$\text{Number of hours} = \text{Specified volume} \div \text{cc/hr}$$

$$\text{Number of hours} = \text{Specified volume} \div \left(\frac{\text{flow rate}}{\text{number of gtt/cc}} \times 60 \right)$$

Which of the two equations you use depends upon the data available. We shall look at examples of both types of computation.

Example

There is 600 cc of intravenous solution. The rate is 75 cc/hr. How many hours will this intravenous last?

To Solve

$$\text{Number of hours} = \text{Specified volume} \div \text{cc/hr}$$
$$= 600 \text{ cc} \div 75 \text{ cc/hr}$$
$$= 8$$

Example

There is 120 cc of fluid left in the intravenous set. The flow rate is 30 gtt/min. How long will this last before a new bottle is needed? (The administration set equivalency is 15 gtt = 1 cc for this example.)

To Solve

$$\text{Number of hours} = \text{Specific volume} \div \left(\frac{\text{flow rate}}{\text{number of gtt/cc}} \times 60 \text{ min} \right)$$

$$= 120 \text{ cc} \div \left(\frac{30 \text{ gtt}}{15 \text{ gtt/cc}} \times 60 \right)$$

$$= 120 \div \left(\frac{\overset{2}{\cancel{30}}}{\underset{1}{\cancel{15}}} \times 60 \right)$$

$$= 120 \div (2 \times 60)$$

$$= 120 \div 120$$

$$= 1$$

► When you feel that you understand this material, complete Activity Sheet 6.

Activity Sheet 6

1. A volume of 2500 cc of fluid is ordered. The patient is to receive 125 cc/hr. It will take _____ hours for the fluid to be administered.

2. You find that there is 360 cc of fluid left. The flow rate is 30 gtt/min. The administration set equivalency is 15 gtt = 1 cc. How long will this fluid last?

3. A volume of 120 cc of fluid is ordered. The patient is to receive 75 cc/hr. It will take _____ hours for the fluid to be administered.

4. You find that there is 120 cc of fluid left. The flow rate is 10 gtt/min. The administration set equivalency is 10 gtt = 1 cc. How long will this fluid last?

5. A volume of 480 cc of fluid is ordered. The patient is to receive 20 cc/hr. It will take _____ hours for the fluid to be administered.

6. You find that there is 150 cc of fluid left. The flow rate is 15 gtt/min. The administration set equivalency is 60 gtt = 1 cc. How long will this fluid last?

7. A volume of 3000 cc of fluid is ordered. The patient is to receive 125 cc/hr. It will take _____ hours for the fluid to be administered.

8. You find that there is 180 cc of fluid left. The flow rate is 45 gtt/min. The administration set equivalency is 15 gtt = 1 cc. How long will this fluid last?

▶ Compare your answers with those at the end of this chapter. If you have answered all questions correctly, continue to the text that follows. Otherwise, review the previous text and correct your mistakes before proceeding.

CALCULATING THE FLUID VOLUME RECEIVED PER HOUR WHEN THE FLUID VOLUME RECEIVED PER MINUTE IS KNOWN

Suppose you know that a person is being given a certain number of cc/min. How do you determine the amount of cc/hr this person is receiving?

Number of cc/hr =
        cc/min × 60 min (number of minutes in 1 hour)

Example

A person is receiving 2.5 cc/min. How many cc/hr is this?

To Solve

Number of cc/hr = cc/min × 60 min

= 2.5 cc/min × 60 min

= 150

▶ When you feel that you understand this material, complete Activity Sheet 7.

Activity Sheet 7

Assuming the following infusion rates, determine the number of cubic centimeters per hour being given.

1. $1\frac{1}{4}$ cc/min = _____ cc/hr

2. $2\frac{1}{3}$ cc/min = _____ cc/hr

3. 3.2 cc/min = _____ cc/hr

4. 1.4 cc/min = _____ cc/hr

5. 2.75 cc/min = _____ cc/hr

► Compare your answers with those at the end of this chapter. If you have answered all questions correctly, continue to the text that follows. Otherwise, review the previous text and correct your mistakes before proceeding.

CALCULATING THE FLUID VOLUME RECEIVED FOR A SPECIFIC FLOW RATE

Suppose that you know a person's infusion is set at a specified number of drops per minute. How would you determine the amount of fluid volume in cubic centimeters that a person is receiving (a) per minute, (b) per hour, and (c) in multiple hours?

$$\text{(a) Number of cc/min} = \frac{\text{Flow rate (gtt/min)}}{\text{Number of gtt/cc}}$$

(b) Number of cc/hr =

$$\frac{\text{Flow rate (gtt/min)}}{\text{Number of gtt/cc}} \times \frac{60 \text{ min}}{\text{(number of minutes in 1 hour)}}$$

or

Number of cc/hr =
    Number of cc/min × 60 min (number of minutes in 1 hour)

(c) Number of cc in multiple hours =

$$\frac{\text{Flow rate (gtt/min)}}{\text{Number of gtt/cc}} \times \frac{60 \text{ min}}{\text{(minutes in 1 hour)}} \times \frac{\text{number of hours}}{\text{fluid is to infuse}}$$

or

Number of cc in multiple hours =
    Number of cc/hr × number of hours fluid is to infuse

Example

An intravenous solution is infused at a flow rate of 15 gtt/min. The administration set equivalency is 10 gtt = 1 cc. Calculate the amount of fluid volume in cubic centimeters that this person is receiving (a) per minute, (b) per hour, and (c) in the 8 hours you will be caring for him or her.

To Solve

(a) Number of cc/min $= \dfrac{\text{Flow rate (gtt/min)}}{\text{Number of gtt/cc}}$

$= \dfrac{15 \text{ gtt/min}}{10 \text{ gtt/cc}}$

$= 1.5 \text{ cc/min}$

(b) Number of cc/hr $= \dfrac{\text{Flow rate (gtt/min)}}{\text{Number of gtt/cc}} \times 60 \text{ min/hr}$

$= \dfrac{15 \text{ gtt/min}}{10 \text{ gtt/cc}} \times 60 \text{ min/hr}$

$= 1.5 \text{ cc/min} \times 60 \text{ min/hr}$

$= 90 \text{ cc/hr}$

(c) Number of cc in multiple hours

$= \dfrac{\text{Flow rate (gtt/min)}}{\text{Number of gtt/cc}} \times 60 \text{ min/hr} \times \begin{matrix} \text{number of hours} \\ \text{fluid is to infuse} \end{matrix}$

$= \dfrac{15 \text{ gtt/min}}{10 \text{ gtt/cc}} \times 60 \text{ min/hr} \times 8 \text{ hr}$

$= 1.5 \text{ cc/min} \times 60 \text{ min/hr} \times 8 \text{ hr}$

$= 720 \text{ cc}$

▶   When you feel that you understand this material, complete Activity Sheet 8.

Activity Sheet 8

1. An infusion has a flow rate of 10 gtt/min. The administration set equivalency is 15 gtt = 1 cc. Calculate the amount of fluid volume in cubic centimeters that a person is receiving (a) per minute, (b) per hour, and (c) in 12 hours.

2. An infusion flow rate is 12 gtt/min. The administration set equivalency is 15 gtt = 1 cc. Calculate the number of cubic centimeters received (a) per minute, (b) per hour, and (c) in 10 hours.

3. Answer the above question for an administration set marked 10 gtt = 1 cc.

4. Given a flow rate of 20 gtt/min and an administration set equivalency 10 gtt = 1 cc, calculate the number of cubic centimeters received (a) per minute, (b) per hour, and (c) in 24 hours.

5. Answer the above question for an administration set marked 15 gtt = 1 cc.

► Compare your answers with those at the end of this chapter. If you have answered all questions correctly, take the posttest. Otherwise, review the previous text and correct your mistakes before taking the posttest.

Posttest

1. What are your mathematical responsibilities with regard to the intravenous administration of fluids?

2. Why may the flow rates of two administrations vary but still deliver the same amount of fluid per hour?

3. Why may the flow rates of two intravenous administrations be identical but deliver different amounts of fluid volume?

4. List four common IV administration set drop equivalencies (that is, the number of drops in 1 cc).

5. Why must you check the literature enclosed in the fluid administration set before you calculate a flow rate?

6. A person is to receive 1200 cc of fluid over 24 hours. How many cc/hr should this person receive?

7. If 2000 cc of fluid is to be absorbed over a 24-hour period, how many cc/hr should be administered?

8. The infusion rate is 180 cc/hr. How many cc/min is this?

9. The infusion rate is 20 cc/hr. How many cc/min is this?

For questions 10 through 14, calculate the flow rates for administration sets having the following equivalencies: (a) 15 gtt = 1 cc, (b) 12 gtt = 1 cc, (c) 10 gtt = 1 cc, and (d) 60 gtt = 1 cc.

10. The infusion rate is 3 cc/min. The flow rates should be
    (a)   (b)
    (c)   (d)

11. The infusion rate is 1 cc/min. The flow rate should be
    (a)   (b)
    (c)   (d)

213

TPO	IPO
1	8,9, or 10

12. The infusion rate is 75 cc/hr. The flow rates should be
    (a)   (b)
    (c)   (d)

1	8,9, or 10

13. The infusion rate is 30 cc/hr. The flow rates should be
    (a)   (b)
    (c)   (d)

1	8,9, or 10

14. If 1200 cc of fluid is to be administered over a 20-hour period, the flow rates should be
    (a)   (b)
    (c)   (d)

1	8,9, or 10

15. If 480 cc of blood is to be administered over a 4-hour period, what infusion rate should be used?

	11

16. The fluid administration rate is 85 cc/hr. How much fluid will be received in 24 hours?

	11

17. If a person receives fluid at a rate of 120 cc/hr for the 8 hours you administer care, he or she should receive _____ cc.

	12

18. If 1500 cc of fluid is ordered, and the patient is to receive 125 cc/hr, it will take _____ hours for the fluid to be administered.

	12

19. If 1800 cc of fluid is ordered, and the patient is to receive 90 cc/hr, it will take _____ hours for the fluid to be administered.

2	12

20. You find that there is 240 cc of fluid left. The flow rate is 30 gtt/min. The administration set equivalency is 10 gtt = 1 cc. How long will this fluid last?

2	12

21. You find that there is 90 cc of fluid left. The flow rate is 60 gtt/min. How long will this fluid last? (The administration set equivalency is 60 gtt = 1 cc.)

2	12

22. You find that there is 100 cc of fluid left. The flow rate is 20 gtt/min. The administration set equivalency is 10 gtt = 1 cc. How long will this fluid last?

	13

23. An infusion instills $1\frac{1}{3}$ cc/min. At this rate, how many cc/hr will be administered?

24. An intravenous flow rate is 45 gtt/min. The administration set equivalency is 15 gtt = 1 cc. Calculate the amount of fluid volume in cubic centimeters that this person is receiving (a) per minute, (b) per hour, and (c) in an 8-hour period.

25. An intravenous flow rate is 90 gtt/min. The administration set equivalency is 60 gtt = 1 cc. Calculate the amount of fluid volume in cubic centimeters that this person is receiving (a) per minute, (b) per hour, and (c) in a 12-hour period.

▶ Compare your answers with those listed at the end of this chapter. If you have answered all questions correctly, begin the next chapter. Otherwise, note the number next to your incorrect test item, return to the relevant text, review it, and practice the appropriate items on the activity sheets. Then correct your mistakes on this test and take the pretest of this chapter as a second posttest, before continuing to the next chapter.

Answers for Chapter 8

PRETEST

1. Calculate (a) the number of cc/hr to administer and (b) the flow rat[e]
   to use.

2,3. Because the drops delivered by the two are of different size.

4. 15 gtt = 1 cc; 12 gtt = 1 cc; 10 gtt = 1 cc; and 60 gtt = 1 cc.

5. To verify the number of drops equal to 1 cc.

6. 150

7. 125

8. 2

9. $\dfrac{1}{6}$

10. (a) 30   (b) 24   (c) 20   (d) 120

11. (a) $7\dfrac{1}{2} \approx 7$ or 8   (b) 6   (c) 5   (d) 30

12. (a) 45   (b) 36   (c) 30   (d) 180

13. (a) $31\dfrac{1}{4} \approx 31$ (b) 25   (c) $20\dfrac{5}{6} \approx 21$ (d) 125

14. (a) 30   (b) 24   (c) 20   (d) 120

15. 25

16. 1920

17. 1000

18. 25

19. 20

20. 2 hours

21. $\dfrac{1}{2}$ hour (30 minutes)

22. $\dfrac{5}{6}$ hour (50 minutes)

23. 90

24. (a) 4   (b) 240   (c) 1920

25. (a) $\dfrac{3}{4}$ (b) 45   (c) 540

ACTIVITY SHEET 1

1. To compute (a) the number of cc/hr to administer and (b) the flow rate to use.
2. The number of drops per minute at which the intravenous is infusing.
3. The number of drops that equals 1 cc.
4,5. Because the drops delivered by each set are of different size.
6. 15 gtt = 1 cc; 12 gtt = 1 cc; 10 gtt = 1 cc; and 60 gtt = 1 cc.
7. To verify the number of drops that equals 1 cc.

ACTIVITY SHEET 2

1. 75

2. 125

3. $41\frac{2}{3}$

4. 100

5. 50

6. $1\frac{1}{4}$

7. $2\frac{1}{12}$

8. $\frac{1}{4}$

9. $1\frac{2}{3}$

10. $\frac{5}{6}$

11. (a) $18\frac{3}{4} \approx 19$ (b) 15   (c) $12\frac{1}{2} \approx 12$ or 13   (d) 75

12. (a) $31\frac{1}{4} \approx 31$ (b) 25   (c) $20\frac{5}{6} \approx 21$ (d) 125

13. (a) $10\frac{5}{12} \approx 10$ (b) $8\frac{1}{3} \approx 8$ (c) $6\frac{17}{18} \approx 7$ (d) $41\frac{2}{3} \approx 42$

14. (a) 25   (b) 20   (c) $16\frac{2}{3} \approx 17$ (d) 100

15. (a) $12\frac{1}{2} \approx 13$ (b) 10   (c) $8\frac{1}{3} \approx 8$ (d) 50

16. (a) 60   (b) 48   (c) 40   (d) 240

17. (a) $22\frac{1}{2} \approx 23$ (b) 18   (c) 15   (d) 90

18. (a) 15   (b) 12   (c) 10   (d) 60

19. (a) 25   (b) 20   (c) $16\frac{2}{3} \approx 17$ (d) 100

20. (a) 30   (b) 24   (c) 20   (d) 120

21. (a) 50   (b) 40   (c) $33\frac{1}{3} \approx 33$ (d) 200

22. (a) $31\frac{1}{4} \approx 31$ (b) 25   (c) $20\frac{5}{6} \approx 21$ (d) 125

23. (a) 25   (b) 20   (c) $16\frac{2}{3} \approx 17$ (d) 100

24. (a) $31\frac{1}{4} \approx 31$ (b) 25   (c) $20\frac{5}{6} \approx 21$ (d) 125

25. (a) $16\frac{2}{3} \approx 17$ (b) $13\frac{1}{3} \approx 13$ (c) $11\frac{1}{9} \approx 11$ (d) $66\frac{2}{3} \approx 67$

26. (a) $15\frac{5}{8} \approx 16$ (b) $12.5 \approx 13$ (c) $10\frac{5}{12} \approx 10$ (d) $62\frac{1}{2} \approx 63$

27. (a) $62\frac{1}{2} \approx 63$ (b) 50   (c) $41\frac{2}{3} \approx 42$ (d) 250

28. $16\frac{2}{3} \approx 17$ 29. $37\frac{1}{2} \approx 38$

30. 20

ACTIVITY SHEET 3

1. (a) $15.6 \approx 16$ (b) $12.5 \approx 13$ (c) $10.4 \approx 10$ (d) $62.5 \approx 63$
2. (a) $20.8 \approx 21$ (b) $16.6 \approx 17$ (c) $13.8 \approx 14$ (d) $83.3 \approx 83$
3. (a) $37.5 \approx 38$ (b) 30   (c) 25   (d) 150
4. (a) $17.5 \approx 18$ (b) 14   (c) $11.6 \approx 12$ (d) 70
5. (a) $12.5 \approx 13$ (b) 10   (c) $8.3 \approx 8$ (d) 50
6. (a) $18.75 \approx 19$ (b) 15   (c) $12.5 \approx 13$ (d) 75
7. (a) $21.25 \approx 21$ (b) 17   (c) $14.2 \approx 14$ (d) 85
8. (a) 10   (b) 8   (c) $6.6 \approx 7$ (d) 40
9. $18.75 \approx 19$
10. $13.3 \approx 13$
11. $18.75 \approx 19$
12. $20.8 \approx 21$
13. $187.5 \approx 188$
14. $83.333 \approx 83$
15. 100

ACTIVITY SHEET 4

1. (a) 4   (b) 5   (c) 6
   (d) 1, or the flow rate equals the number of cc/hr
2. (a) cc/hr ÷ 4 = flow rate   (b) cc/hr ÷ 5 = flow rate
   (c) cc/hr ÷ 6 = flow rate   (d) cc/hr = flow rate

3. (a) $12\frac{1}{2} \approx 13$ (b) 10   (c) $8\frac{1}{3} \approx 8$ (d) 50

4. (a) $18\frac{3}{4} \approx 19$ (b) 15   (c) $12\frac{1}{2} \approx 13$ (d) 75

5. (a) $6\frac{1}{4} \approx 6$ (b) 5   (c) $4\frac{1}{6} \approx 4$ (d) 25

6. (a) 10   (b) 8   (c) $6\frac{2}{3} \approx 7$ (d) 40

7. (a) 15   (b) 12   (c) 10   (d) 60

8. (a) $22\frac{1}{2} \approx 23$ (b) 18   (c) 15   (d) 90

9. (a) 36   (b) $28.8 \approx 29$ (c) 24   (d) 144

10. (a) 30   (b) 24   (c) 20   (d) 120

11. 15   12. 20

13. (a) 3   (b) 40   14. (a) 10   (b) 15

ACTIVITY SHEET 5

1. 1500   2. 2640   3. 2100   4. 600   5. 640

ACTIVITY SHEET 6

1. 20   2. 3 hours   3. 1.6 hours (1 hour 36 minutes)
4. 2 hours   5. 24   6. 10 hours
7. 24   8. 1 hour

ACTIVITY SHEET 7

1. 75   2. 140   3. 192   4. 84   5. 165

ACTIVITY SHEET 8

1. (a) $\frac{2}{3}$ (b) 40   (c) 480   2. (a) $\frac{4}{5}$ (b) 48   (c) 480

3. (a) 1.2 $\left(1\frac{1}{5}\right)$ (b) 72   (c) 720

4. (a) 2   (b) 120   (c) 2880

5. (a) $1\frac{1}{3}$ (b) 80   (c) 1920

POSTTEST

1. To calculate (a) the number of cc/hr to administer and (b) the flow rate to use

2,3. Because the drops delivered by the two sets are of different size

4. 15 gtt = 1 cc; 12 gtt = 1 cc; 10 gtt = 1 cc; 60 gtt = 1 cc

5. To verify the number of drops that equals 1 cc

6. 50

7. $83\dfrac{1}{3}$

8. 3

9. $\dfrac{1}{3}$

10. (a) 45   (b) 36   (c) 30   (d) 180

11. (a) 15   (b) 12   (c) 10   (d) 60

12. (a) $18\dfrac{3}{4} \approx 19$ (b) 15   (c) $12\dfrac{1}{2} \approx 13$ (d) 75

13. (a) $7\dfrac{1}{2} \approx 8$ (b) 6   (c) 5   (d) 30

14. (a) 15   (b) 12   (c) 10   (d) 60

15. 20

16. 2040

17. 960

18. 12

19. 20

20. $1\dfrac{1}{3}$ hours (1 hour 20 minutes)

21. $1\dfrac{1}{2}$ hours (1 hour 30 minutes)

22. $\dfrac{5}{6}$ hour (50 minutes)

23. 80

24. (a) 3   (b) 180   (c) 1440

25. (a) $1\dfrac{1}{2}$ (b) 90   (c) 1080

9 | *Mathematical Aspects of the Administration of Intravenous Medications*

1. Given a prescribed medication dosage a person is to receive in a specific fluid volume during a specified time interval, the reader is able to calculate the flow rate at which to set the infusion.
2. Given a prescribed dosage a person is to receive per minute and the amount of medication in a certain fluid volume, the reader is able to calculate the flow rate at which to set the infusion.
3. Given a prescribed dosage a person is to receive per kilogram of body weight per minute and the amount of medication in a certain fluid volume, the reader is able to calculate the flow rate at which to set the infusion.
4. Given the flow rate and the amount of medication in a certain volume, the reader is able to compute the amount of medication a person is receiving per minute.
5. Given the flow rate and the amount of medication in a specified volume, the reader is able to compute the amount of medication per kilogram of body weight a person is receiving per minute.
6. Given a prescribed dosage a person is to receive per hour and the amount of medication in a certain fluid volume, the reader is able to calculate the flow rate at which to set the infusion.
7. Given the flow rate and the amount of medication in a specified volume, the reader is able to calculate the amount of medication a person is receiving per hour.

221

INTERMEDIATE PERFORMANCE OBJECTIVES

After studying the text, the reader is able to:

1. State the physician's responsibility with regard to intravenous medications for patients.
2. State the nurse's responsibility with regard to intravenous medications for patients.
3. List the four items of information that must be collected to enable the nurse to safely and accurately perform her mathematical responsibilities with regard to the administration of intravenous medications.
4. State an additional piece of information that must be obtained from the literature for intravenous medications to be administered properly.
5. List the drop equivalencies (drop factors) for the four most commonly used fluid administration sets.
6. List the special number for each of the four most common fluid administration sets that when divided into the number of cc/hr a person is to receive will give you the flow rate (gtt/min) at which to set the infusion.
7. Compute the amount of fluid to be administered per hour.
8. Calculate the concentration per cubic centimeter of a solution being administered.
9. State the flow rate that delivers 1 cc/min for the set being used.
10. State the fluid administration set equivalency that is used most frequently for the infusion of intravenous medications.
11. Explain the rationale for using the set referred to in Intermediate Performance Objective 10.

▶ If you feel confident that you possess these skills, take the pretest that follows. Otherwise, begin to study the material in this chapter.

Pretest

For questions 1 through 5 calculate the flow rate at which to set the infusion.

1. Prescribed dose: 500 mcg
   Specified dilution: 75 cc
   Specified infusion time interval: $\frac{1}{2}$ hour
   Administration set equivalency: 60 gtt = 1 cc

2. Prescribed dose: 3 g
   Specified dilution: 120 cc
   Specified infusion time interval: 2 hours
   Administration set equivalency: 10 gtt = 1 cc

3. Prescribed dose: 1,000,000 U
   Specified dilution: 100 cc
   Specified infusion time interval: 15 minutes
   Administration set equivalency: 15 gtt = 1 cc

4. Prescribed dose: 750 mg
   Specified dilution: 90 cc
   Specified infusion time interval: $\frac{3}{4}$ hour
   Administration set equivalency: 60 gtt = 1 cc

5. Prescribed dose: 30,000 U
   Specified dilution: 50 mL
   Specified infusion time interval: 20 minutes
   Administration set equivalency: 12 gtt = 1 cc

For questions 6 through 15 calculate the flow rate for the situation; for each item the administration set equivalency is 60 gtt = 1 cc.

6. A medicated intravenous solution is labeled 200 mg per 250 cc. The person is to receive 240 mcg/min of this medication.

TPO	IPO
2	8,9
2	8,9
2	8,9
2	8,9
3	8,9
3	8,9
3	8,9
3	8,9
3	8,9
4	8,9
4	8,9
4	8,9

7. An intravenous mixture is labeled 400 U per 250 mL. The person is to receive 1.2 U/min of this medication.

8. A medicated intravenous solution labeled as an 8:1 concentration contains 1.6 g per 200 cc. The person is to receive 3 mg/min of this medicine.

9. A medicated intravenous solution is labeled 500 mg/L. The person is to receive 0.375 mg/min of this medicine.

10. A medicated intravenous solution is labeled 0.8 g/L. The person is to receive 200 mcg/min of this medicine.

11. Medicated intravenous solution: 450 mg per 500 cc
Person's weight: 60 kg
Prescribed dose: 6 mcg/kg/min

12. Intravenous mixture: 14,000 U per 250 cc
Person's weight: 154 lb
Prescribed dose: 0.4 U/kg/min

13. Medicated intravenous solution: 450 mg per 0.5 L
Person's weight: 132 lb
Prescribed dose: 10 mcg/kg/min

14. Intravenous mixture: 2.8 g/L
Person's weight: 70 kg
Prescribed dose: 0.02 mg/kg/min

15. Medicated intravenous solution: 0.32 g per 500 cc
Person's weight: 80 kg
Prescribed dose: 4 mcg/kg/min

16. There is 200 mg of medication in 125 ml of intravenous fluid. The flow rate is 12 microgtt/min. The administration set equivalency is 60 gtt = 1 cc. How many micrograms of medication is this person receiving per minute?

17. There is 20,000 U of medication in 500 cc of intravenous fluid. The flow rate is 15 pedigtt/min. The administration set equivalency is 60 gtt = 1 cc. How many units of medication is this person receiving per minute?

18. There is 4 mg of medication in 500 mL of intravenous fluid. The flow rate is 30 minigtt/min. The administration set equivalency is

TPO   IPO

60 gtt = 1 cc. How many micrograms of medication is this person receiving per minute?

4   8,9   19. There is 250 mg of medication in 500 cc of intravenous fluid. The flow rate is 15 microgtt/min. The administration set equivalency is 60 gtt = 1 cc. How many milligrams of medication is this person receiving per minute?

4   8,9   20. There is 60,000 U of medication in 1 L of intravenous fluid. The flow rate is 55 microgtt/min. The administration set equivalency is 60 gtt = 1 cc. How many units of medication is this person receiving per minute?

For questions 21 through 25, calculate the amount of medication per kilogram of body weight per minute a person is receiving in the measurement indicated. The administration set equivalency is 60 gtt = 1 cc.

5   8,9   21. Medicated intravenous solution: 450 mg per 500 cc
Person's weight: 50 kg
Flow rate: 15 microdrips/min
Number of mcg/kg/min: _____

5   8,9   22. Intravenous mixture: 21,000 U/500 cc
Person's weight: 110 lb
Flow rate: 20 microdrips/min
Number of U/kg/min: _____

5   8,9   23. Medicated intravenous solution: 900 mg/1 L
Person's weight: 45 kg
Flow rate: 15 microdrips/min
Number of mcg/kg/min: _____

5   8,9   24. Intravenous mixture: 0.75 g/1 L
Person's weight: 50 kg
Flow rate: 20 microdrips/min
Number of mcg/kg/min: _____

5   8,9   25. Medicated intravenous solution:
3 g/1000 cc (3:1 concentration, 3 mg/cc)
Person's weight: 45 kg
Flow rate: 18 microdrips/min
Number of mcg/kg/min: _____

6   7   26. Medicated intravenous solution: 60,000 U/1 L
Administer: 600 U/hr
Infusion rate: _____ cc/hr

TPO	IPO
6	7

27. Medicated intravenous solution: 500 mg per 500 cc D5W
Administer: 50 mg/hr
Infusion rate: _____ cc/hr

TPO	IPO
6	7

28. Medicated intravenous solution: 100 U per 500 cc NS
Administer: 4 U/hr
Infusion rate: _____ cc/hr

TPO	IPO
6	7

29. Medicated intravenous solution: 10 mg per 100 cc
Administer: 3 mg/hr
Infusion rate: _____ cc/hr

TPO	IPO
6	7

30. Medicated intravenous solution: 25,000 U per 500 cc
Administer: 150 U/hr
Infusion rate: _____ cc/hr

TPO	IPO
7	7

31. Medicated intravenous solution: 50 mg per 500 cc D5W
Infusion rate: 25 cc/hr
Dosage per hour is _____ mg

TPO	IPO
7	7

32. Medicated intravenous solution: 25 mg per 250 cc NS
Infusion rate: 5 cc/hr
Dosage per hour: _____ mg

TPO	IPO
7	7

33. Medicated intravenous solution: 30,000 U per 500 cc D5W
Infusion rate: 9 cc/hr
Dosage per hour: _____ U

TPO	IPO
7	7

34. Medicated intravenous solution: 50,000 U per 500 cc
Infusion rate: 45 cc/hr
Dosage per hour: _____ U

TPO	IPO
7	7

35. Medicated intravenous solution: 20 mg/200 cc
Infusion rate: 50 cc/hr
Dosage per hour: _____ mg

▶ Compare your answers with those at the end of this chapter. If you have answered all questions correctly, begin the next chapter. Otherwise, begin this chapter by reading the next section of text.

GENERAL INFORMATION

With increasing frequency medications are given intravenously. Normally the physicians will prescribe the dosage of medication to be given and the nurse will be responsible for preparing and administering the medication dosage. This chapter is designed to provide you with sufficient practice to be able to perform the mathematical calculations necessary to fulfill this responsibility.

In your practice you will find that the administration prescription of intravenous drugs varies. A prescribed dose may be given as a direct push bolus of a medication. In this situation you may be injecting as little as $\frac{1}{2}$ to 1 cc of a drug directly into a vein without further dilution.

Intravenous medications are also first diluted and then administered periodically or intermittently over a specified time interval. This method is employed, for example, in the administration of antibiotics, antihypertensives, or other such drugs when the intravenous route is necessary for a better therapeutic effect or when the person is unable to take medication orally. In this method you would take the prescribed medication (e.g., 250 mg), dilute it in a certain amount of solution (e.g., 100 cc), and administer it over a certain time interval (e.g., 30 minutes). This method of administering intravenous medications is often called "piggyback IV med" (for reasons that the figure below should make obvious). The person receiving the intravenous medication already has a mainline (primary set) of solution running. A second medication can be administered intermittently by connecting it (via a secondary set) into the infusion that has already been established. The diagram on page 228 illustrates this procedure.

The third method of intravenous administration of medications is continuous infusion. It involves placing a prescribed dose (e.g., 500 mg) in a prescribed solution (e.g., 500 cc D5W) and running it at a prescribed rate (e.g., 20 mg/hr or 20 cc/hr). Typical medications given by this method are aminophylline and heparin.

From the above paragraphs you should realize that your responsibilities go far beyond a mathematical aspect; we did not even begin to talk about the knowledge you must possess relative to the action of the drug. Although knowledge of drug action is not the focus of this book we would be remiss if we did not emphasize strongly enough how important it is that you *consult available current literature and keep up to date and knowledgeable about both the drug and its administration.*

This text emphasizes the mathematical aspect of administering drugs; to perform your responsibilities in this area safely and accurately, you must collect the following data:

1. With how much intravenous fluid volume must this dose be diluted before administration?

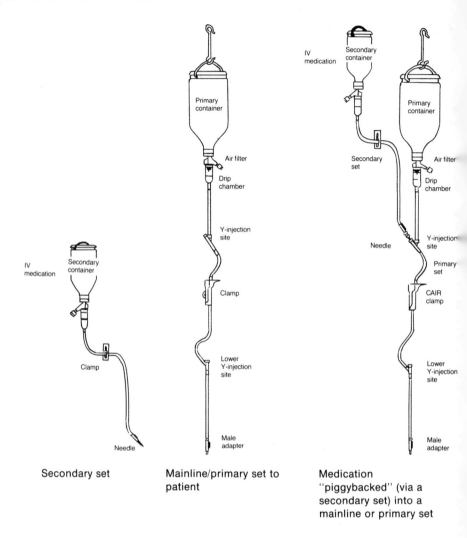

Secondary set

Mainline/primary set to patient

Medication "piggybacked" (via a secondary set) into a mainline or primary set

2. During what time interval must the fluid volume be administered?

3. How many drops equal 1 cc for the administration set used?

4. What special number should be utilized for the available administration set?

There are a number of other responsibilities you will have with regard to the administration of intravenous solutions, however. You will need to consult the literature to determine the type of intravenous solution that may be used to dilute a prescribed medication. Drug compatibility—

both with other drugs and with varied intravenous solutions—is also of critical importance: some drug combinations are incompatible; others are unstable. If a person has other drugs running or a solution that is not compatible with the drug you now want to give you must formulate an alternative plan for administering the drug. Lastly, you must be very careful with the infusion rate or time—even as little as 1 cc may have a prescribed amount of time over which it must be given (e.g., give drug over 5 minutes). *Always read the available literature carefully.*

CALCULATING FLOW RATES FOR INTERMITTENT DILUTED BOLUS MEDICATIONS (PIGGYBACK IV MEDS)

As discussed in the previous chapter, the equivalencies for the four most common fluid administration sets are as follows:

1. 15 gtt = 1 cc
2. 12 gtt = 1 cc
3. 10 gtt = 1 cc
4. 60 gtt = 1 cc

The 60-gtt/cc set is used for the slow administration of fluids and is especially useful when an infusion pump is unavailable, as it prevents the medicated solution from being instilled too rapidly.

The "special numbers" for fluid administration sets (also discussed in the previous chapter) are as follows:

Fluid Administration Set	Special Number
1 cc = 15 gtt	4
1 cc = 12 gtt	5
1 cc = 10 gtt	6
1 cc = 60 gtt	1

Example

Prescribed dose: 500 mg of an antibiotic

Specified dilution (or the amount of intravenous fluid volume in which the medication is to be contained): 50 cc

Specified infusion time interval: 30 minutes

Administration set equivalency: 15 gtt = 1 cc

Flow rate: _____ gtt/min

To Solve

The formula method presented in chapter 8 calculates the flow rate (gtt/min) by means of the following equation:

$$\text{Flow rate} = \frac{\text{Fluid volume} \times \text{number of gtt/cc}}{\text{Time in minutes}}$$

Substituting the values from the example into this equation, we obtain

$$\text{Flow rate} = \frac{50 \text{ cc} \times 15 \text{ gtt/cc}}{30 \text{ min}}$$

$$= \frac{50 \times \overset{1}{\cancel{15}}}{\underset{2}{\cancel{30}}}$$

$$= \frac{\overset{25}{\cancel{50}} \times 1}{\underset{1}{\cancel{2}}}$$

$$= \frac{25 \times 1}{1}$$

$$= 25 \text{ gtt/min}$$

Example

Medication order 80 mg IV
Literature reference:

Dose	Dilution	Administration Time
50 mg	50 cc D5W	30–60 min
>50 mg	100 cc D5W	1 hour

Administration sets available on your unit: 60 gtt = 1 cc
10 gtt = 1 cc

To Solve

This problem can be solved using either the formula method or the short method illustrated in chapter 8 by means of the following equation:

Flow rate = cc/hr ÷ "special number"

If you use the 10 gtt = 1 cc administration set the special number will be 6 and the flow rate will be

$$\text{Flow rate} = 100 \div 6$$

$$= 16\frac{2}{3} \approx 17 \text{ gtt/min}$$

If you use the 60 gtt = 1 cc administration set, the special number will be 1 and the flow rate will be

$$\text{Flow rate} = 100 \div 1$$

$$= 100 \text{ gtt/min}$$

Because the special number of an administration set with an equivalency of 60 gtt = 1 cc is 1, the flow rate (gtt/min) is the same as the infusion rate (cc/hr), and the equation can be solved in one step:

$$100 \text{ cc/hr} = 100 \text{ gtt/min}$$

Please note: In some problems the flow rate is very high, for example, 300 gtt/min, if you use the microdrop set (60 gtt = 1 cc). Because it is impossible to count such a number and be accurate, you should use one of the other administration sets.

▶ When you feel that you understand this material, complete Activity Sheet 1.

Activity Sheet 1

1. What is the physician's responsibility with regard to intravenous medications for patients?

2. What is the nurse's responsibility with regard to intravenous medications for patients?

3. To perform the mathematical nursing responsibilities for the safe and accurate administration of intravenous drugs, what four items of information must be collected?

4. What additional essential item of information must be gathered from the literature to administer medications intravenously?

5. List the drop equivalencies for the four most commonly used fluid administration sets.

6. List the special numbers for the four most common fluid administration sets.

For questions 7 through 16 calculate the flow rate.

7. Prescribed dose: 1 g
   Specified dilution: 240 cc
   Specified time interval: 1 hour
   Administration set equivalency: 10 gtt = 1 cc

8. Prescribed dose: 80 mg
   Specified dilution: 200 cc
   Specified time interval: 2 hours
   Administration set equivalency: 15 gtt = 1 cc

9. Prescribed dose: 500 mg
   Specified dilution: 50 cc
   Specified time interval: $\frac{1}{2}$ hour (30 minutes)
   Administration set equivalency: 60 gtt = 1 cc

10. Prescribed dose: 250 mg
    Specified dilution: 25 cc
    Specified time interval: 1 hour
    Administration set equivalency: 60 gtt = 1 cc

11. Prescribed dose: 1,000,000 U
    Specified dilution: 180 cc
    Specified time interval: 2 hours
    Administration set equivalency: 10 gtt = 1 cc

12. Prescribed dose: 0.5 g
    Specified dilution: 100 cc
    Specified time interval: $\frac{1}{2}$ hour (30 minutes)
    Administration set equivalency: 15 gtt = 1 cc

13. Prescribed dose: 40 mg
    Specified dilution: 150 cc
    Specified time interval: 2 hours
    Administration set equivalency: 60 gtt = 1 cc

14. Prescribed dose: 50 mg
    Specified dilution: 500 cc
    Specified time interval: 6 hours
    Administration set equivalency: 15 gtt = 1 cc

15. Prescribed dose: 2 g
    Specified dilution: 150 cc
    Specified time interval: $\frac{1}{2}$ hour (30 minutes)
    Administration set equivalency: 10 gtt = 1 cc

16. Prescribed dose: 90 mg
    Specified dilution: 150 cc
    Specified time interval: $1\frac{1}{2}$ hours (90 minutes)
    Administration set equivalency: 60 gtt = 1 cc

17. Prescribed dose: 300 mg
    Specified dilution: 50 cc
    Specified time interval: 15 minutes
    Administration set equivalency: 12 gtt = 1 cc

18. Prescribed dose: 600 mg
    Specified dilution: 100 cc
    Specified time interval: 20 minutes
    Administration set equivalency: 12 gtt = 1 cc

19. Prescribed dose: 500 mg
    Specified dilution: 250 cc
    Specified time interval: 45 minutes
    Administration set equivalency: 15 gtt = 1 cc

20. Prescribed dose: 1 g
    Specified dilution: 100 cc
    Specified time interval: 15 minutes
    Administration set equivalency: 12 gtt = 1 cc

▶ Compare your answers with those at the end of this chapter. If you have answered all questions correctly, continue to the text that follows. Otherwise, review the previous text and correct your mistakes before continuing.

MATHEMATICAL ASPECTS FOR THE ADMINISTRATION OF CONTINUOUS MEDICATED SOLUTIONS—PRESCRIBED PER MINUTE

Very frequently patients receive medications via continuous intravenous infusion. In these situations the physician's order generally consists of (1) the name and amount of medication, (2) the amount and type of solution in which it is to be mixed, and (3) the dosage the person is to receive, for example, lidocaine 2 g in 500 cc of D5W run it at 3 mg/min. In some situations the physician may only write the name of the medication and the amount the patient is to receive (i.e., administer lidocaine at 3 mg/min). You and/or institutional policy may determine the dilution of this medication prior to its administration. Note that the medication prescription in this example is to be administered per minute but other such prescriptions may be administered per hour. In all these situations to administer the prescribed dose you must calculate the intravenous flow rate. The examples and activity sheets that follow should provide you with sufficient practice to master this skill. Although you may be able to use any type of fluid administration set in this calculation, you will find that it is best to use a set that delivers 60 gtt/cc because the small drop size will provide a means for ensuring the slow administration of a medicated fluid volume.

Guide to Solve

Step 1: Find the drug concentration per cc.

> Concentration/cc =
>   Total amount of medication ÷ total fluid volume

Be sure that the levels of measurement here is the same as that of the prescribed dose, i.e., g, mg, or mcg.

Step 2: State the flow rate that delivers 1 cc/min for the set being used. The set equivalency corresponds to the flow rate that would deliver 1 cc/min:

Set Equivalency	Flow Rate → 1 cc/min
15 gtt = 1 cc	15 gtt/min
12 gtt = 1 cc	12 gtt/min
10 gtt = 1 cc	10 gtt/min
60 gtt = 1 cc	60 gtt/min (set most often used)

Step 3: Compute the flow rate.

$$\frac{\text{Concentration of drug per cc}}{\substack{\text{Flow rate that delivers} \\ \text{1 cc/min for the set used}}} = \frac{\text{Prescribed dose/min}}{\substack{x\,(\text{Flow rate at which} \\ \text{to set the infusion})}}$$

The first relationship can be established because if you know, for example, that 20 mg is in every 1 cc (20 mg/cc) and the equivalency of the administration set is 60 gtt = 1 cc, it is the same as saying 20 mg is in 60 gtt:

$$\frac{20 \text{ mg}}{1 \text{ cc}} \text{ is the same as } \frac{20 \text{ mg}}{60 \text{ gtt}}$$

In the box above, x is the flow rate required to deliver the prescribed amount of medication per minute.

Example

Administration set utilized: 60 gtt = 1 cc
Medicated intravenous solution: 2 g per 500 cc
Prescribed dose: 3 mg/min

To Solve
We must first convert the 2 g per 500 cc solution to the same level of the metric system as the prescribed dose (3 mg/min). To convert 2 g to milligrams we multiply by 1000: 2 g = 2000 mg.

Step 1: Find the drug concentration per cc.

$$\text{Concentration/cc} = \\ \text{Total amount of medication} \div \text{total fluid volume}$$

$$\text{Concentration/cc} = 2000 \text{ mg} \div 500 \text{ cc}$$

$$= \frac{2000 \text{ mg}}{500 \text{ cc}} = \frac{4 \text{ mg}}{1 \text{ cc}}$$

$$= 4 \text{ mg/cc}$$

Step 2: State the flow rate that delivers 1 cc/min for the set being used. Since the set equivalency is 60 gtt = 1 cc,

Flow rate of 60 gtt/min delivers 1 cc/min.

Step 3: Compute the flow rate.

$$\frac{\text{Concentration of drug per cc}}{\begin{array}{c}\text{Flow rate that delivers}\\ \text{1 cc/min for the set used}\end{array}} = \frac{\text{Prescribed dose/min}}{\begin{array}{c}x \text{ (Flow rate at which}\\ \text{to set the infusion)}\end{array}}$$

$$\frac{4 \text{ mg}^a}{60 \text{ gtt/min}} = \frac{3 \text{ mg}}{x}$$

$$4x = 3 \times 60$$

$$4x = 180$$

$$x = 45 \text{ gtt/min}$$

^{a} Remember step 1 and that concentration 4 mg/cc is the same as 4 mg/60 gtt (because 60 gtt = 1 cc).

► When you feel that you understand this material, complete Activity Sheet 2.

Activity Sheet 2

1. State the mathematical responsibility you will have that is mentioned in the previous section of text in regard to the administration of intravenous medications.

2. What fluid administration set is used most frequently for the infusion of intravenous medications? Why?

3. State the flow rate that delivers 1 cc/min for the following administration set equivalencies:
   (a) 15 gtt = 1 cc
   (b) 12 gtt = 1 cc
   (c) 10 gtt = 1 cc
   (d) 60 gtt = 1 cc

For questions 4 through 11 calculate (a) the concentration per cc and (b) the flow rate. For all of these situations assume that the administration set equivalency is 60 gtt = 1 cc.

4. A mixed intravenous fluid is labeled as 400 mg per 250 cc. The person is to receive 400 mcg/min of this medication.

5. An intravenous mixture is labeled as 200 U per 250 cc. The person is to receive 0.2 U/min.

6. An intravenous mixture labeled as a 3:1 concentration contains 600 mg per 200 cc. The person is to receive 0.75 mg/min.

7. An intravenous mixture is labeled as 2 g per 200 cc. The person is to receive 4 mg/min.

8. An intravenous solution is labeled as 200 mg per 500 mL. The patient is to receive an initial dose of 140 mcg/min.

9. An intravenous mixture is labeled as 100 U/250 mL. A patient is to receive 0.2 U/min.

10. A medicated intravenous solution is labeled as 2 g per 250 cc. A patient is to receive 6 mg/min.

11. A medicated intravenous solution is labeled as 0.8 g per 500 cc. A patient is to receive 1200 mcg/min.

12. The medicated intravenous solution is labeled 8 mg per 500 cc. The patient is to receive 8 mcg/min.

13. The medicated intravenous solution is 4 g per 500 cc and the patient is to receive 4 mg/min.

▶ Compare your answers with those at the end of this chapter. If you have answered all questions correctly, continue to the text that follows. Otherwise, review the previous text and correct your mistakes before continuing.

MATHEMATICAL ASPECTS FOR THE ADMINISTRATION OF CONTINUOUS MEDICATED SOLUTIONS—PRESCRIBED ACCORDING TO BODY WEIGHT

In certain situations the amount of medications to be administered via continuous intravenous infusion depends upon the weight of the individual. The steps to calculate the flow rate in these instances are the same as were discussed in the previous section:

Step 1: Find the concentration of drug per cc.

Step 2: State the flow rate that delivers 1 cc/min for the set being used.

Step 3: Compute the flow rate.

Example

Calculate the flow rate that will deliver the prescribed dose in the following situation:

Medicated intravenous solution: 225 mg per 250 cc
Person's weight: 132 lb (60 kg)
Prescribed dose: 3 mcg/kg/min
Administration set equivalency: 60 gtt = 1 cc

To Solve

Step 1: Calculate the concentration per cc of the solution being administered. Since the prescribed dose is in micrograms, we first convert the medicated intravenous solution into micrograms: 225 mg = 225,000 mcg.

> Concentration/cc =
>   Total amount of medication ÷ total fluid volume

Concentration/cc = 225,000 mcg ÷ 250 cc

= 900 mcg/cc

Step 2: State the flow rate (gtt/min) that delivers 1 cc/minute for the set being utilized. The set equivalency is 60 gtt = 1 cc, so

Flow rate of 60 gtt/min delivers 1 cc/min

Step 3: Compute the flow rate.

$$\frac{\text{Concentration of drug per cc}}{\substack{\text{Flow rate that delivers} \\ \text{1 cc/min for the set used}}} = \frac{\text{Prescribed dose/min}}{\substack{x\,(\text{Flow rate at which} \\ \text{to set the infusion})}}$$

This is where the calculation differs from that of the previous example. Before we can solve the equation, we must first compute the amount of medication that is to be received per minute. This is easily done using the following formula:

Prescribed dose/min = Amount of medication/kg/min

$$\times \text{ number of kg of body weight}$$

$$= 3 \text{ mcg} \times 60$$

$$= 180 \text{ mcg}$$

We use this result in the flow rate computation as follows:

$$\frac{900 \text{ mcg}}{60 \text{ gtt}} = \frac{3 \text{ mcg/kg/min or } 180 \text{ mcg/min}}{x}$$

$$900x = 180 \times 60$$

$$900x = 10,800$$

$$x = 10,800 \div 900$$

$$= 12 \text{ gtt/min}$$

► When you feel that you understand this material, complete Activity Sheet 3.

Activity Sheet 3

1. List the steps that you would use to calculate the flow rate for a continuously infused dosage of medication per minute that is prescribed on the basis of a person's weight.

2. Write the equation (step 3 of question 1) that you will use to calculate the flow rate for these type of problems.

3. How would you calculate what the prescribed dose of medication per minute should be?

For questions 4 through 9, calculate the flow rate necessary to administer the prescribed dose. Assume that the administration set equivalency is 60 gtt = 1 cc.

4. Medicated intravenous solution: 450 mg per 500 cc
   Person's weight: 90 kg
   Prescribed dose: 3 mcg/kg/min

5. Intravenous mixture: 14,000 U per 250 cc
   Person's weight: 154 lb
   Prescribed dose: 0.2 U/kg/min

6. Medicated intravenous solution: 450 mg per 0.5 L
   Person's weight: 132 lb
   Prescribed dose: 7.5 mcg/kg/min

7. Intravenous mixture: 2.8 g/L
   Person's weight: 70 kg
   Prescribed dose: 0.01 mg/kg/min

8. Medicated intravenous solution: 0.48 g per 750 cc
   Person's weight: 80 kg
   Prescribed dose: 4 mcg/kg/min

9. Intravenous mixture: 0.12 g/L
   Person's weight: 176 lb
   Prescribed dose: 0.1 mcg/kg/min

▶ Compare your answers with those at the end of this chapter. If you have answered all questions correctly, continue to the text that follows. Otherwise, review the previous text and correct your mistakes before continuing.

CALCULATING THE AMOUNT OF MEDICATION A PERSON IS RECEIVING WHEN THE FLOW RATE IS KNOWN

Another situation may arise in the clinical area that will require additional mathematical skills: you may know (1) the amount of medication contained in a specified volume of fluid, (2) the fluid administration set equivalency, and (3) the flow rate at which an infusion is set, but may be asked or want to know (a) the amount of medication the patient is being administered per minute and/or (b) the amount of medication per kilogram of body weight being administered per minute. In the text that follows, you should note that the steps involved in solving these questions are the same as those used in the previous two sections, the difference lying in which is the unknown quantity.

Before you begin your calculations, be sure that the medication quantities identified in the problem are in the same system of measurement and also at the same level of measurement within the same system. If they are not, convert the larger unit to the smaller unit of measurement.

Guide to Solve

Step 1: Calculate the concentration/cc (amount of medication/cc) of solution being administered.

> Concentration/cc =
>   Total amount of medication ÷ total fluid volume

Step 2: State the flow rate that equals 1 cc for the set being used.

Step 3: Compute the amount of medication administered per minute for a given flow rate.

$$\frac{\text{Concentration of drug per cc}}{\substack{\text{Flow rate that delivers}\\ \text{1 cc/min for the set used}}} = \frac{x\,(\text{Medication/minute})}{\substack{\text{Flow rate at which}\\ \text{infusion is set}}}$$

Here x is the amount of medication administered per minute. The following is the computation to use when it is necessary to know the amount of medication per kilogram of body weight administered per minute:

$$\text{Amount of medication/kg/min} =$$

$$\frac{\text{Amount of medication administered per minute}}{\text{Kilograms of body weight}}$$

Example

Intravenous medication label: 400 mg per 250 cc
Flow rate: 20 gtt/min
Administration set equivalency: 60 gtt = 1 cc
Body weight: 40 kg
How many micrograms per minute is the patient receiving?
How many micrograms per kilogram of body weight is the patient receiving?

To Solve

1. Inspect the medication quantities in the problem. Ask yourself:
   (a) Are these measurements in the same system? Yes. (b) Are these measurements at the same level? No. Because 400 mg is one level of measurement and micrograms is another, we convert 400 mg into micrograms:

   $$\frac{1 \text{ mg}}{1000 \text{ mcg}} = \frac{400 \text{ mg}}{x}$$

   $$x = 400 \times 1000$$

   $$x = 400{,}000 \text{ mcg}$$

   Therefore, we can express the concentration as 400,000 mcg per 250 cc.
2. Calculate the concentration of medication/cc.

Concentration/cc =
  Total amount of medication ÷ total fluid volume

$$\text{Concentration/cc} = 400{,}000 \text{ mcg} \div 250 \text{ cc}$$

$$= 1600 \text{ mcg/cc}$$

3. Compute the amount of medication administered per minute for a given flow rate.

$$\frac{\text{Concentration of drug per cc}}{\substack{\text{Flow rate that delivers} \\ \text{1 cc/min for the set used}}} = \frac{x\,(\text{Medication/minute})}{\substack{\text{Flow rate at which} \\ \text{infusion is set}}}$$

$$\frac{1600\ \text{mcg}}{60\ \text{gtt/min}} = \frac{x\,(\text{mcg/min})}{20\ \text{gtt}}$$

$$60x = 20 \times 1600$$

$$60x = 32,000$$

$$x = 533\frac{1}{3}\ \text{mcg/min}$$

4. Computation when it is necessary to know the amount of medication per kilogram of body weight administered per minute.

$$\text{Amount of medication/kg/min} = \frac{\text{Amount of medication administered/min}}{\text{Number of kilograms of body weight}}$$

$$\text{Amount of medication/kg/min} = \frac{533\frac{1}{3}\ \text{mcg/min}}{40\ \text{kg}}$$

$$= 533\frac{1}{3} \div 40$$

$$= \frac{1600}{3} \div 40$$

$$= \frac{1600}{3} \times \frac{1}{40}$$

$$= 13\frac{1}{3}\ \text{mcg/kg/min}$$

▶ When you feel that you understand this material, complete Activity Sheet 4.

Activity Sheet 4

1. There is 0.8 g of medication in 500 cc of intravenous fluid. The flow rate is 45 gtt/min. the administration set equivalency is 60 gtt = 1 cc. How many micrograms of medication is this person receiving per minute?

2. There is 4 g of medication in 500 cc of intravenous fluid. The flow rate is 15 gtt/min. The administration set equivalency is 60 gtt = 1 cc. How many milligrams of medication is this person receiving per minute?

3. There is 400 U of medication in 500 cc of intravenous fluid. The flow rate is 45 gtt/min. The administration set equivalency is 60 gtt = 1 cc. How many units of medication is this person receivng per minute?

4. There is 200 mg of medication in 125 cc of intravenous fluid. The flow rate is 24 gtt/min. The administration set equivalency is 60 gtt = 1 cc. How many micrograms of medication is the person receiving per minute?

5. There is 40,000 U of medication in 1000 mL of intravenous fluid. The flow rate is 36 gtt/min. The administration set equivalency is 60 gtt = 1 cc. How many units of medication is this person receiving per minute?

6. There is 4 mg of a medication in 1 L of intravenous fluid. The flow rate is 15 gtt/min. The administration set equivalency is 60 gtt = 1 cc. How many micrograms of medication is this person receiving per minute?

7. There is 35,000 U of medication in 1 L of intravenous fluid. The flow rate is 12 gtt/min. The administration set equivalency is 60 gtt = 1 cc. How many units of medication is this person receiving per minute?

8. There is an 8:1 preparation (8 mg/cc) presently infusing. The flow rate is 10 gtt/min. The administration set equivalency is 60 gtt = 1 cc. How many milligrams of medication is this person receiving per minute?

9. There is 30,000 U of medication in 750 cc of intravenous fluid. The flow rate is 48 gtt/min. The administration set equivalency is 60 gtt = 1 cc. How many units of medication is this person receiving per minute?

10. There is a 3:1 preparation (3 mg/cc) presently infusing. The flow rate is 40 gtt/min. The administration set equivalency is 60 gtt = 1 cc. How many milligrams per minute is this person receiving?

For questions 11 through 13, calculate the amount of medication per kilogram of body weight per minute a person is receiving:

11. Medicated intravenous solution: 450 mg per 500 cc
Person's weight: 60 kg
Flow rate: 12 gtt/min
Administration set equivalency: 60 gtt = 1 cc
Amount of mcg/kg/min: _____

12. Intravenous mixture: 42,000 U per 1000 cc
Person's weight: 77 lb
Flow rate: 30 gtt/min
Administration set equivalency: 60 gtt = 1 cc
Amount of U/kg/min: _____

13. Medicated intravenous solution: 900 mg per 0.75 L
Person's weight: 80 kg
Flow rate: 45 gtt/min
Administration set equivalency: 60 gtt = 1 cc
Amount of mcg/kg/min: _____

▶ Compare your answers with those at the end of this chapter. If you have answered all questions correctly, continue to the text that follows. Otherwise, review the previous text and correct your mistakes before continuing.

CALCULATING FLOW RATE FOR THE ADMINISTRATION OF A PRESCRIBED AMOUNT OF MEDICINE PER HOUR

At times you will need to calculate the flow rate that will administer a prescribed dosage of medication per hour (rather than per minute, as was discussed in the previous section), for example, during the administration of continuous heparin or aminophylline. In these situations the physician usually writes an order such as "mix 30,000 U of heparin in 500 cc D5W and administer 840 U/hr." The process for calculating the flow rates in these situations is in actuality easier than the previous problems we have practiced. The mathematical calculations you will perform to administer such a prescribed dose, as you will note, is to calculate the amount of cubic centimeters per hour to administer.

Usually these continuous medicated solutions are administered via some type of infusion pump. The pumps you will encounter have settings where they infuse cubic centimeters per hour or microgtts per minute. As was shown previously, if the administration set has an equivalency of 60 gtt = 1 cc, the number of drops per minute is the same as the number of cubic centimeters per hour; thus, if we decide to run 25 cc/hr, we would set the flow rate at 25 gtt/min. The same applies here. Once you have calculated the number of cc/hr the person must receive to obtain the prescribed dose, you have figured out at which number to set either a pump or an IV.

Example

Medicated solution: 30,000 U in 500 cc D5W
Infusion rate: 840 U/hr
At what should you set the infusion rate?
Flow rate: _____ cc/hr (or gtt/min)

To Solve
First find the amount of solution that contains the prescribed dose.

$$\frac{\text{Total amount medication}}{\text{Total fluid volume (cc)}} = \frac{\text{Prescribed dose}}{x \text{ (Fluid amount)}}$$

$$\frac{30{,}000 \text{ U}}{500 \text{ cc}} = \frac{840 \text{ U}}{x \text{ (cc)}}$$

$$\frac{\overset{60}{\cancel{30{,}000}} \text{ U}}{\underset{1}{\cancel{500}}} = \frac{840 \text{ U}}{x \text{ (cc)}}$$

$$\frac{60 \text{ U}}{1 \text{ cc}} = \frac{840 \text{ U}}{x \text{ (cc)}}$$

$$60x = 840 \text{ cc}$$

$$x = 840 \div 60$$

$$x = 14 \text{ cc}$$

Answer to Problem
14 cc. If this fluid amount is administered per hour from this particular IV bottle containing 30,000 U/500 cc, the person would receive 840 U of medication (the prescribed dose). To administer this amount IV (14 cc/hr):

Set the microdrop unit at 14 gtt/min

or

Set the infusion pump at 14 cc/hr

▶ When you feel that you understand this material, complete Activity Sheet 5.

Activity Sheet 5

1. If you had to administer 50 cc/hr and you were using a microdrop fluid administration set (60 gtt = 1 cc), what flow rate would you use?

2. When a prescribed dose is to be administered per hour, what is the guide this section suggests you use to solve this problem?

For questions 3 through 12, calculate the flow rate in cc/hr and gtt/min to administer the prescribed dose.

3. Medicated intravenous solution: 500 mg per 500 cc D5W
   Prescribed dose: 40 mg/hr

4. Medicated intravenous solution: 10,000 U per 100 cc D5W
   Prescribed dose: 700 U/hr

5. Medicated intravenous solution: 25 mg per 250 cc NS
   Prescribed dose: 2 mg/hr

6. Medicated intravenous solution: 30,000 U per 500 cc D5W
   Prescribed dose: 960 U/hr

7. Medicated intravenous solution: 100 U per 500 cc NS
   Prescribed dose: 6 U/hr

8. Medicated intravenous solution: 50 mg per 500 cc D5W
   Prescribed dose: 5 mg/hr

9. Medicated intravenous solution: 50,000 U per 500 cc NS
   Prescribed dose: 1000 U/hr

10. Medicated intravenous solution: 10 mg per 100 cc D5W
    Prescribed dose: 1 mg/hr

11. Medicated intravenous solution: 25,000 U per 500 cc NS
    Prescribed dose: 1200 U/hr

12. Medicated intravenous solution: 30,000 U/L NS
    Prescribed dose: 600 U/hr

▶   Compare your answers with those at the end of this chapter. If you have answered all
    questions correctly, continue to the next section of text. Otherwise, review the previous
    text and correct your mistakes before continuing.

CALCULATING THE AMOUNT OF MEDICATION BEING RECEIVED PER HOUR WHEN THE FLOW RATE IS KNOWN

You may be faced with a situation where a patient has a continuous medicated solution being administered (e.g., 60,000 U/L), you know the infusion rate (e.g., 15 cc/hr)—for that is at what the infusion pump is set, and you want to verify both that the patient is receiving the correct dosage of medication and that this dosage lies within the safety range for that particular drug.

Example

Medicated solution: 60,000 U in 1 L D5W
Infusion pump rate: 15 cc/hr
Total dosage: _____ U/hr

To Solve

To calculate this problem we shall use the same guide discussed in the previous section of text.

$$\frac{\text{Total amount of medication}}{\text{Total amount of fluid (cc)}} = \frac{x \text{ (prescribed dose)}}{\text{Fluid amount (cc/hr)}}$$

Reduce to

$$\frac{60,000 \text{ U}}{1000 \text{ cc}} = \frac{x \text{ U}}{15 \text{ cc/hr}}$$

$$\frac{60 \text{ U}}{1 \text{ cc}} = \frac{x \text{ U}}{15 \text{ cc/hr}}$$

$$x = 60 \times 15$$

$$x = 900 \text{ U/hr}$$

Thus, if there is 60,000 U of medication in 1 L of fluid, the person receives 900 U/hr when the infusion rate is 15 cc/hr.

Example

Medicated solution: 60,000 U in 1 L D5W
Flow rate: 30 gtt/min
Administration set equivalency: 60 gtt = 1 cc
Total dosage: _____ U/hr

To Solve

$$\frac{\text{Total amount of medication}}{\text{Total amount of fluid (cc)}} = \frac{x \text{ (prescribed dose)}}{\text{Fluid amount (cc/hr)}}$$

Because the administration set equivalency is 60 gtt = 1 cc, if the flow rate is 30 gtt/min, the infusion rate is 30 cc/hr. We now substitute the other variables into the equation:

$$\frac{60,000 \text{ U}}{1000 \text{ cc}} = \frac{x \text{ (U)}}{30 \text{ cc/hr}}$$

Reduce to

$$\frac{60 \text{ U}}{1 \text{ cc}} = \frac{x \text{ (U)}}{30 \text{ cc/hr}}$$

$$x = 60 \times 30$$

$$x = 1800 \text{ U/hr}$$

Thus, a person receiving 30 gtt/min of solution (30 cc/hr) is receiving 1800 U/hr of medication.

▶   When you feel that you understand this material, complete Activity Sheet 6.

Activity Sheet 6

For questions 1 through 10 calculate the amount of medication a person is receiving per hour where administration set equivalency is 60 gtt = 1 cc.

1. Medicated intravenous solution: 500 mg per 500 cc D5W
   Flow rate: 25 cc/hr

2. Medicated intravenous solution: 10,000 U per 100 cc D5W
   Flow rate: 12 gtt/min

3. Medicated intravenous solution: 25 mg per 250 cc D5W
   Flow rate: 25 cc/hr

4. Medicated intravenous solution: 30,000 U per 500 cc D5W
   Flow rate: 17 cc/hr

5. Medicated intravenous solution: 100 U per 500 cc NS
   Flow rate: 60 gtt/min

6. Medicated intravenous solution: 50 mg per 500 cc D5W
   Flow rate: 45 cc/hr

7. Medicated intravenous solution: 50,000 U per 500 cc NS
   Flow rate: 15 gtt/min

8. Medicated intravenous solution: 10 mg per 100 cc
   Flow rate: 12 cc/hr

9. Medicated intravenous solution: 25,000 U per 500 cc NS
   Flow rate: 30 cc/hr

10. Medicated intravenous solution: 30,000 U/L NS
    Flow rate: 19 gtt/min

▶ Compare your answers with those at the end of this chapter. If you have answered all questions correctly, continue to the Posttest. Otherwise, review the previous text and correct your mistakes before continuing.

Posttest

<table>
<tr><td>TPO</td><td>IPO</td><td></td></tr>
<tr><td></td><td></td><td>For questions 1 through 5 calculate the flow rate at which to set the infusion:</td></tr>
</table>

For questions 1 through 5 calculate the flow rate at which to set the infusion:

1. Prescribed dose: 125 mcg
   Specified dilution: 25 cc
   Specified infusion time interval: 30 minutes
   Administration set equivalency: 60 gtt = 1 cc

2. Prescribed dose: 2.5 g
   Specified dilution: 225 mL
   Specified infusion time interval: 3 hours
   Administration set equivalency: 10 gtt = 1 cc

3. Prescribed dose: 1,200,000 U
   Specified dilution: 200 cc
   Specified infusion time interval: 20 minutes
   Administration set equivalency: 15 gtt = 1 cc

4. Prescribed dose: 250 mg
   Specified dilution: 80 mL
   Specified infusion time interval: 40 minutes
   Administration set equivalency: 60 gtt = 1 cc

5. Prescribed dose: 4000 U
   Specified dilution: 50 cc
   Specified infusion time interval: 15 minutes
   Administration set equivalency: 12 gtt = 1 cc

   For questions 6 through 15 calculate the flow rate; assume that the administration set equivalency is 60 gtt = 1 cc.

6. A medicated intravenous solution is labeled 200 mg per 250 cc. The person is to receive 120 mcg/min of this medicine.

7. A medicated intravenous solution is labeled 400 U per 250 mL. The person is to receive 0.4 U/min of this medicine.

TPO	IPO	
2	8,9	**8.** A medicated intravenous solution labeled as an 8:1 concentration contains 1.6 g per 200 cc. The person is to receive 1 mg/min of this medicine.
2	8,9	**9.** A medicated intravenous solution is labeled 500 mg/L. The person is to receive 0.125 mg/min of this medicine.
2	8,9	**10.** A medicated intravenous solution is labeled 0.8 g/L. The person is to receive 600 mcg/min of this medicine.
3	8,9	**11.** Medicated intravenous solution: 450 mg per 500 cc Person's weight: 60 kg Prescribed dose: 1.5 mcg/kg/min
3	8,9	**12.** Intravenous mixture: 28,000 U per 500 cc Person's weight: 154 lb Prescribed dose: 0.4 U/kg/min
3	8,9	**13.** Medicated intravenous solution: 450 mg per 0.5 L Person's weight: 132 lb Prescribed dose: 5 mcg/kg/min
3	8,9	**14.** Intravenous mixture: 5.6 g/L Person's weight: 70 kg Prescribed dose: 0.04 mg/kg/min
3	8,9	**15.** Medicated intravenous solution: 0.32 g per 500 cc Person's weight: 80 kg Prescribed dose: 2 mcg/kg/min
4	8,9	**16.** There is 200 mg of medication in 125 mL of intravenous fluid. The administration set equivalency is 60 gtt = 1 cc and the flow rate is 48 gtt/min. How many micrograms of medication is this person receiving per minute?
4	8,9	**17.** There is 20,000 U of medication in 0.5 L of intravenous fluid. The administration set equivalency is 60 gtt = 1 cc and the flow rate is 45 gtt/min. How many units of medication is this person receiving per minute?
4	8,9	**18.** There is 4 mg of medication in 500 cc of intravenous fluid. The administration set equivalency is 60 gtt = 1 cc and the flow rate is 15 gtt/min. How many micrograms of medication is this person receiving per minute?

TPO	IPO
4	8,9
4	8,9
5	8,9
5	8,9
5	8,9
5	8,9
5	8,9

19. There is 250 mg of medication in 500 cc of intravenous fluid. The administration set equivalency is 60 gtt = 1 cc and the flow rate is 45 gtt/min. How many milligrams of medication is this person receiving per minute?

20. There is 50,000 U of medication in 1 L of intravenous fluid. The administration set equivalency is 60 gtt = 1 cc and the flow rate is 15 gtt/min. How many units of medication is this person receiving per minute?

For questions 21 through 25, calculate the amount of medication per kilogram of body weight per minute a person is administered in the measurement indicated.

21. Medicated intravenous solution: 225 mg per 250 cc
Person's weight: 75 kg
Flow rate: 20 gtt/min
Administration set equivalency: 60 gtt = 1 cc
Number of mcg/kg/min: _____

22. Intravenous mixture: 90,000 U per 250 cc
Person's weight: 99 lb
Flow rate: 15 gtt/min
Administration set equivalency: 60 gtt = 1 cc
Number of U/kg/min: _____

23. Medicated intravenous solution: 750 mg per 0.25 L
Person's weight: 40 kg
Flow rate: 10 gtt/min
Administration set equivalency: 60 gtt = 1 cc
Number of mcg/kg/min: _____

24. Intravenous mixture: 0.25 g/L
Person's weight: 100 kg
Flow rate: 30 gtt/min
Administration set equivalency: 60 gtt = 1 cc
Number of mcg/kg/min: _____

25. Medicated intravenous solution: 8 g per 1000 cc
Person's weight: 80 kg
Administration set equivalency: 60 gtt = 1 cc
Flow rate: 12 gtt/min
Number of mcg/kg/min: _____

PO	IPO

26. Medicated intravenous solution: 60,000 U/L NS
Administer: 1200 U/hr
Flow rate: _____ cc/hr

27. Medicated intravenous solution: 500 mg per 500 cc D5W
Administer: 35 mg/hr
Flow rate: _____ cc/hr

28. Medicated intravenous solution: 100 U per 500 cc NS
Administer: 15 U/hr
Flow rate: _____ cc/hr

29. Medicated intravenous solution: 10 mg per 100 cc D5W
Administer: 1.5 mg/hr
Flow rate: _____ cc/hr

30. Medicated intravenous solution: 25,000 U per 500 cc NS
Administer: 900 U/hr
Flow rate: _____ cc/hr

31. Medicated intravenous solution: 50 mg per 500 cc D5W
Infusion rate: 35 cc/hr
Dosage per hour: _____ mg

32. Medicated intravenous solution: 25 mg per 250 cc NS
Infusion rate: 28 cc/hr
Dosage per hour: _____ mg

33. Medicated intravenous solution: 30,000 U per 500 cc D5W
Infusion rate: 20 cc/hr
Dosage per hour: _____ U

34. Medicated intravenous solution: 50,000 U per 500 cc NS
Infusion rate: 18 cc/hr
Dosage per hour: _____ U

35. Medicated intravenous solution: 20 mg per 200 cc NS
Infusion rate: 36 cc/hr
Dosage per hour: _____ mg

► Compare your answers with those listed at the end of this chapter. If you have answered all questions correctly, begin the next chapter. Otherwise, note the number next to the item(s) you answered incorrectly, return to the relevant text, review it, and practice the appropriate items on the activity sheets. Then recalculate the items you answered incorrectly on this test and take the pretest of this chapter as a second posttest before continuing to the next chapter.

The PO/IPO column values for items 26–35:

Item	PO	IPO
26		7
27		7
28		7
29	6	7
30	6	7
31	7	7
32	7	7
33	7	7
34	7	7
35	7	7

Answers for Chapter 9

PRETEST

1. 150	2. 10	3. 100
4. 120	5. 30	6. 18
7. 45	8. $22\frac{1}{2} \approx 23$	9. 45
10. 15	11. 24	12. 30
13. 40	14. 30	15. 30
16. 320	17. 10	18. 4
19. 0.125	20. 55	21. 4.5
22. 0.28	23. 5	24. 5
25. 20	26. 10	27. 50
28. 20	29. 30	30. 3
31. 2.5	32. 0.5	33. 540
34. 4500	35. 5	

ACTIVITY SHEET 1

1. Prescription of the medication dosage
2. Preparation and administration of the medication
3. (a) In how much intravenous fluid volume must this dose be diluted?
   (b) In what specified time interval must the fluid volume be administered?
   (c) How many drops equal 1 cc for the administration set utilized?
   (d) What "special number" should be used for the available administration set?
4. The type of intravenous fluid that should be utilized to dilute the specific medication
5. 1 cc = 15 gtt, 1 cc = 12 gtt, 1 cc = 10 gtt, 1 cc = 60 gtt
6. 4, 5, 6, 1

7. 40	8. 25	9. 100
10. 25	11. 15	12. 50

260

13. 75	14. $20.8 \approx 21$	15. 50
16. 100	17. 40	18. 60
19. 83	20. 80	

ACTIVITY SHEET 2

1. To calculate the intravenous flow rate to ensure that the patient is receiving a prescribed amount of medication per minute
2. A set with the equivalency 60 gtt = 1 cc because it provides for the safer administration of medications by allowing fluids to flow at a slower rate
3. (a) 15gtt/min   (b) 12 gtt/min   (c) 10 gtt/min
   (d) 60 gtt/min
4. (a) 1600 mcg   (b) 15
5. (a) 0.8 U   (b) 15
6. (a) 3 mg   (b) 15
7. (a) 10 mg   (b) 24
8. (a) 400 mcg   (b) 21
9. (a) 0.4 U   (b) 30
10. (a) 8 mg   (b) 45
11. (a) 1600 mcg   (b) 45
12. (a) 16 mcg   (b) 30
13. (a) 8 mg   (b) 30

ACTIVITY SHEET 3

1. Step 1: Find the concentration of drug per cc.
   Step 2: State the flow rate that delivers 1 cc/min for the set being used.
   Step 3: Compute the flow rate.
2. $$\frac{\text{Concentration of drug per cc}}{\text{Flow rate that delivers 1 cc for the set used}} = \frac{\text{Prescribed dose/min}}{x \,(\text{Flow rate, gtt/min})}$$
3. Prescribed dose per minute = Amount of medication/kg/min $\times$ kg of body weight

4. 18	5. 15	6. 30
7. 15	8. 30	9. 4

ACTIVITY SHEET 4

1. 1200	2. 2	3. 0.6
4. 640	5. 24	6. 1
7. 7	8. $1\frac{1}{3}$	9. 32
10. 2	11. 3	12. 0.6
13. 11.25		

ACTIVITY SHEET 5

1. 50 gtt/min

2. $$\frac{\text{Total amount medication}}{\text{Total fluid volume (cc)}} = \frac{\text{Prescribed dose}}{x \text{ (cc) (Fluid amount)}}$$

	cc/hr	gtt/min
3.	40	40
4.	7	7
5.	20	20
6.	16	16
7.	30	30
8.	50	50
9.	10	10
10.	10	10
11.	24	24
12.	20	20

ACTIVITY SHEET 6

1. 25 mg	2. 1200 U	3. 2.5 mg
4. 1020 U	5. 12 U	6. 4.5 mg
7. 1500 U	8. 1.2 mg	9. 1500 U
10. 570 U		

POSTTEST

1. 50

2. $12\frac{1}{2} \approx 13$

3. 150

4. 120

5. 40

6. 9

7. 15

8. $7\frac{1}{2} \approx 8$

9. 15

10. 45

11. 6

12. 30

13. 20

14. 30

15. 15

16. 1280

17. 30

18. 2

19. 0.375

20. 12.5

21. 4

22. 2

23. 12.5

24. 1.25

25. 20

26. 20

27. 35

28. 75

29. 15

30. 18

31. 3.5

32. 2.8

33. 1200

34. 1800

35. 3.6

10 | *Pediatric Dosages*

TERMINAL PERFORMANCE OBJECTIVES

1. Given a child's weight and a prescribed amount of medication per pound or kilogram, the reader is able to calculate the dosage to be administered.
2. Given a child's body surface area and a recommended dose per square meter or an average adult dose, the reader is able to calculate the dose to be administered.
3. The reader is able to calculate a child's or infant's dosage using either Freid's, Clark's, or Young's rule.
4. Given the necessary data, the reader is able to calculate the intravenous flow rate to administer prescribed dosages over a specified time interval.
5. Given the necessary data, the reader is able to calculate the intravenous flow rate to administer a prescribed dosage of medication per minute.
6. Given the necessary data, the reader is able to calculate the intravenous flow rate to administer a prescribed dosage of medication per hour.
7. Given the necessary data, the reader is able to compute the number of cubic centimeters or tablets to be administered for a prescribed dose.
8. Given the necessary data, the reader is able to calculate the administration of the infant's or child's dose in household measures.

INTERMEDIATE PERFORMANCE OBJECTIVE

After studying the text the reader is able to state a prime reason why nurses should know how to calculate drug dosages for infants and children.

▶   If you feel that you possess these skills, take the pretest that follows. Otherwise, begin to study the material in this chapter.

Pretest

TPO   IPO

1. Why must you be able to calculate infant's and children's dosages accurately and be able to recognize unusual dosage amounts?

1,7

2. Child's weight: 25 kg
   Recommended dose: 0.01 mg/kg
   Medication available: 0.5 mg per 2 cc
   The child's dose should be _____ mg.
   You will give therefore _____ cc.

1,7

3. Child's weight: 44 lb
   Recommended dose: 60 mcg/kg
   Medication available: 1 mg/cc
   The child's dose should be _____ mcg.
   You will give therefore _____ cc.

1,7

4. Child's weight: 40 kg
   Recommended dose: 75 U/kg
   Medication available: 5000 U/cc
   The child's dose should be _____ U.
   You will give therefore _____ cc.

1,7

5. Child's weight: 45 kg
   Recommended dose: 0.1 mg/lb
   Medication available: 3 mg/cc
   The child's dose should be _____ mg.
   You will give therefore _____ cc.

1,7

6. Child's weight: 88 lb
   Recommended dose: 20 μg/kg
   Medication available: 2 mg/cc
   The child's dose should be _____ μg.
   You will give therefore _____ cc.

2

7. Body surface: 0.9 m^2
   Prescribed dose: 750 mg/m^2/day
   The child should receive _____ mg/day.

TPO	IPO
2	

8. Body surface: 1.2 m²
   Prescribed dose: 250 mg/m² every 8 hours
   The child should receive _____ mg every 8 hours.

| 2 | |

9. Body surface: 0.8 m²
   Average adult dose: 1000 mcg
   The child should receive _____ mcg.

| 2 | |

10. Body surface: 1.15 m²
    Average adult dose: 500 mg
    The child should receive _____ mg.

| 3,8 | |

11. (a) A baby is 1 month old. The average adult dose is 0.45 g. The baby should receive _____ mg.
    (b) If the medication available is 1 mg/t, how much will you give in household measures?

| 3,8 | |

12. (a) If a child weighs 50 lb and the average adult dose is 0.24 g, the child should receive _____ mg.
    (b) If the medicine is available as 40 mg per 1/2 oz, you will give _____ T.

| 3,8 | |

13. (a) A child is 4 years old. The average adult dose is 0.24 g. The child should receive _____ mg.
    (b) If the medicine is available as 0.36 g per 2 T, you will administer _____ t.

| 4 | |

14. Solution administration set: 15 gtt = 1 cc
    Child's weight: 35 kg
    Recommended dose:
        1.7–3.5 mg/kg per 24 hours in four to six divided doses
    Prescribed dose: 20 mg in 50 cc D5W every 4 hours
    Administration time: 30 minutes
    Does this prescribed dose appear to be a safe dosage level?
    What should the flow rate be to administer this dose?

| 4 | |

15. Administration equivalency set: 60 gtt = 1 cc
    Child's size: 0.9 m²
    Recommended dose: 250 mg/m² every 8 hours
    Prescribed dose: 225 mg in 75 cc NS every 8 hours
    Administration time: 45 minutes
    Does this prescribed dose appear to be safe?
    What should be the flow rate to administer this dose?

TPO   IPO

For questions 16 through 21 the administration set equivalency is 60 gtt = 1 cc.

5

16. Medicated solution: 5 g per 100 cc
    Recommended dosage: No faster than 50 mg/min
    Prescribed dose: 37.5 mg/min
    The flow rate to administer the prescribed dose is _____ .

5

17. Medicated solution: 12 g per 200 cc D5W
    Recommended dosage: No greater than 60 mg/min
    Prescribed dose: 15 mg/min
    The flow rate to administer the prescribed dose is _____ .

5

18. Medicated solution: 0.4 g per 200 cc
    Recommended dosage: 20–40 mcg/kg/min
    Child's weight: 40 kg
    Prescribed dose: 30 mcg/kg/min
    The flow rate to administer the prescribed dose is _____

5

19. Medicated solution: 0.7 g per 1000 cc
    Recommended dosage: 20–40 mcg/kg/min
    Child's weight: 77 lb
    Prescribed dose: 20 mcg/kg/min
    The flow rate to administer the prescribed dose is _____ .

6

20. Medicated solution: 250 mg per 250 cc
    Child's weight: 50 kg
    Prescribed dose: 0.9 mg/kg/hr
    How much medication per hour should the child receive?
    What should the flow rate be set at to administer this?
    How many cc/hr will this child receive?

6

21. Medicated solution: 200 mg per 250 cc
    Child's weight: 40 kg
    Prescribed dose: 0.5 mg/kg/hr
    How much medication per hour will the child receive?
    What is the flow rate to administer this?
    How many cc/hr will this child receive?

▶ Compare your answers with those at the end of this chapter. If you have answered all questions correctly, go on to chapter 11. Otherwise, begin to study the material in this chapter.

GENERAL INFORMATION

During the administration of medications to pediatric clients your primary mathematical responsibility remains basically what it is for adult clients—to calculate the amount of medication (tablets, pills, capsules, or fluid volume) to be administered for a prescribed dose and to determine the flow rate to be used for intravenous medications. The physician normally prescribes the drug and dosage the pediatric client will receive. In prescribing drugs and their dosage there are some important considerations to be taken into account. An example is the age of the client—certain drugs cannot be prescribed for neonates and very young infants because their liver and kidneys are not fully developed. Another important aspect to consider is the fact that drug metabolism/excretion in children appears to correlate with their body surface area. Lastly, the weight of an individual must be taken into account. The fact that you will be dealing with very small dosages mandates that your calculations be precise for client safety.

With a review of literature through the years in respect to the methods used to calculate a prescribed dosage, one finds that there appears to have been a change in the methods employed to calculate a prescribed pediatric dosage. Although, as I mentioned previously, the aspect of calculating the prescribed dose is in most instances the responsibility of the physician, the person administering the prescribed dose has a professional and legal responsibility to ensure that it does not exceed the recommended safety range for that medication. We will have adequate practice in this area to ensure that you become comfortable with these calculations.

The methods most frequently used to calculate a prescribed dosage (and thus verify that a prescribed dosage lies within the safety range) are based upon the client's body weight or body surface area. These are the principal focus of this chapter. Although not emphasized, the client's age is also sometimes considered in dosage calculations. The other areas covered in this chapter are calculating the amount of medication (tablets, capsules, fluid volume) to be administered for a prescribed dose and calculating flow rates for intravenous medications.

So that your knowledge base will be complete in regard to pediatric dosages this chapter also includes practice with the formulas (Freid's rule, Clark's rule, and Young's rule) that were previously the primary methods of calculating pediatric dosages. You also should be aware of two other formulas (Cowling's and Dilling's Rule), but no practice situations are provided with them, as they are rarely seen. All of these formulas calculated the pediatric dose as a fractional amount of the adult dose.

PEDIATRIC DOSAGES BASED ON WEIGHT

Example

Weight: 44 lb
Recommended amount of a drug: 6 mg/kg of body weight
Drug available: 250 mg per 10 cc

Determine the dosage the child should be given and the amount of fluid to be used in administering this dosage.

Child's dose =
        Body weight in kg × amount of medication/kg body weight
or
Child's dose =
        Body weight in lb × amount of medication/lb body weight

---

1. Calculate the dosage to be given.

As the recommended dosage is given in mg/kg, we begin by converting the child's weight to kilograms.

$$\text{Wt in kg} = \text{Wt in lb} \div 2.2$$
$$= 44 \div 2.2$$
$$= 20$$

Substituting 20 kg into the formula given in the box above, we obtain

Child's dose = Body wt in kg × amount of medication/kg of body wt
$$= 20 \text{ kg} \times 6 \text{ mg/kg}$$
$$= 120 \text{ mg}$$

2. Calculate the amount of fluid to be given to administer the 120 mg.

Available drug (Known ratio) = Prescribed dose (Unknown ratio)

$$\frac{\text{Amount of medication}}{\text{Fluid volume}} = \frac{\text{Amount of medication}}{x \text{ (Fluid volume)}}$$

$$\frac{250 \text{ mg}}{10 \text{ cc}} = \frac{120 \text{ mg}}{x \text{ (cc)}}$$

$$250x = 10 \times 120$$
$$x = 1200 \div 250$$
$$x = 4.8 \text{ cc}$$

▶ When you feel that you understand and have memorized these data, complete Activity Sheet 1.

Activity Sheet 1

For questions 1 through 10, calculate (a) the appropriate safe child's dose to administer and (b) the amount of tablets, pills, capsules, or fluid volume to administer that prescribed dose:

1. Child's weight: 25 lb
   Recommended dose: 1 mg/lb per 24 hours in two divided doses
   Medication available: 25 mg per tablet

2. Child's weight: 30 kg
   Recommended dose: 0.45 mg/kg
   Medication available: 3 mg/mL

3. Child's weight: 45 lb
   Recommended dose: 0.1 mg/lb
   Medication available: 3 mg/mL

4. Child's weight: 20 kg
   Recommended dose: initial dose—70 mcg/kg
   Medication available: 1 mg/cc

5. Child's weight: 77 lb
   Recommended dose: 0.02 mg/kg
   Medication available: 0.5 mg per 2 cc

6. Child's weight: 88 lb
   Recommended dose: 80 U/kg every 4 hours
   Medication available: 1000 U/cc

7. Child's weight: 32 kg
   Recommended dose: 0.1 mL/kg
   Medication available: as a liquid without a concentration (i.e., mg/mL) given

8. Child's weight: 40 kg
   Recommended dose: 20 μg/kg
   Medication available: 2 mg/cc

9. Child's weight: 99 lb
   Recommended dose: 100 U/kg
   Medication available: 5000 U/cc

10. Child's weight: 40 kg
    Recommended dose: 0.01 mL/kg
    Medication available: as a liquid preparation without a concentration given

▶ Compare your answers with those at the end of this chapter. If you have answered all questions correctly, continue to the next section of text. Otherwise, review the text and correct your mistakes before proceeding.

DOSAGES BASED UPON BODY SURFACE AREA

There are two methods for calculating drug dosages using body surface area. Which one you select will probably be determined by what information is available to you. Sometimes the literature accompanying the drug will state the recommended dosage of a drug per square meter (m^2) of an individual (m^2—square meter—being the body surface measurement used). At other times you will use a formula based on body surface measurement and the recommended average adult dose.

Regardless of which method is used, you must know how to determine the body surface area of the individual. This is done by using a chart (see the figure below) called a nomogram. For children of normal height and weight, the central squared-in section can be used: alongside the weight in pounds, the surface area in square meters is given. If you have any question as to a child's being of average size, however, find the height of the individual (in the leftmost column) and the weight (in the rightmost column) and then connect these two points with a straight line. Where this line intersects the surface area column is the surface area (m^2) of that individual. The following will give you examples of two methods followed by practice problems. (Practice on plotting to find the child's surface area on the West nomogram is not provided.)

Example

Body surface area: 0.9 m^2
Recommended dose: 750 mg/m^2 in three divided doses
What should a pediatric client receive per dose?

Pediatric dose = Child's size in m^2 × recommended dose/m^2

$$\text{Pediatric dose} = 0.9 \text{ m}^2 \times 750 \text{ mg/m}^2$$

$$= 675 \text{ mg} \qquad \text{(This is the total dose per day.)}$$

$$\text{Individual dose} = \text{Total dose} \div \text{number of doses}$$

$$= 675 \text{ mg} \div 3$$

$$= 225 \text{ mg each}$$

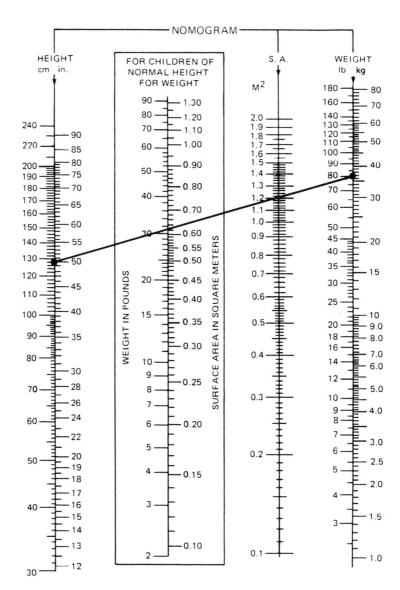

The West nomogram for body surface area. From Behrman, R. E., and Vaughan, V. C. *Nelson Textbook of Pediatrics*, 13th ed. Philadelphia; Saunders, 1987.

Example

Body surface area: 0.9 m²
Average adult dose: 500 mg
What is the pediatric dose?

Pediatric dose =

$$\frac{\text{Surface area of the child in m}^2}{\text{Surface area of average adult in m}^2 \ (= 1.73)} \times \begin{array}{l}\text{average}\\\text{adult dose}\end{array}$$

$$\text{Pediatric dose} = \frac{0.9 \text{ m}^2}{1.73 \text{ m}^2} \times 500 \text{ mg}$$

$$= \frac{450}{1.73}$$

$$= 260.12 \approx 260 \text{ mg}$$

▶ When you feel that you understand and have memorized these data, complete Activity Sheet 2.

Activity Sheet 2

In questions 1 through 8, calculate the pediatric dosage that is safe to administer:

1. Body surface area: 0.8 m^2
   Recommended dose: 750 mg/m^2/day

2. Body surface area: 0.75 m^2
   Average adult dose: 600 mg

3. Body surface area: 0.75 m^2
   Recommended dose: 250 mg/m^2 every 8 hours

4. Body surface area: 0.75 m^2
   Average adult dose: 750 mg

5. Body surface area: 1.1 m^2
   Recommended dose: 250 mg/m^2 three times daily

6. Body surface area: 1.0 m^2
   Average adult dose: 500 mg

7. Body surface area: 1.3 m^2
   Recommended dose: 750 mg/m^2 per 24 hours

8. Body surface area: 1.25 m^2
   Average adult dose: 125 mg

▶ Compare your answers with those at the end of this chapter. If you have answered all questions correctly, proceed to the next section of text. Otherwise, review the text and correct your mistakes before continuing.

FORMULAS USED FOR CALCULATING PEDIATRIC DOSAGES

Listed below are the three major formulas that were used most frequently in the past for the calculation of pediatric dosages. You should be aware of them and be able to follow them if there ever is a need.

Freid's Rule

$$\text{Infant's dose} = \frac{\text{Age (in months)}}{\text{Average adult weight (150 lb)}} \times \text{average adult dose}$$

Clark's Rule

$$\text{Child's dose} = \frac{\text{Weight of child (in pounds)}}{\text{Average adult weight (150 lb)}} \times \text{average adult dose}$$

Young's Rule

$$\text{Child's dose} = \frac{\text{Age of child (in years)}}{\text{Age of child (in years)} + 12} \times \text{average adult dose}$$

Even though you are not likely to use them, and you need not memorize them, you should recognize that other formulas did exist for the calculation of pediatric dosages. Here are two examples:

Cowling's Rule

$$\text{Child's dose} = \frac{\text{Age (in years on next birthday)}}{24} \times \text{average adult dose}$$

Dilling's Rule:

$$\text{Child's dose} = \frac{\text{Age (in years)}}{20} \times \text{average adult dose}$$

Practice is provided only of Freid's rule, Clark's rule, and Young's rule.

Example

Infant's age: 6 months
Average adult dose: 75 mg
How much medication should this baby receive?
If the medication comes as 1.5 mg/t, how much fluid volume in household measure should this baby receive?

To Solve
Freid's rule:

$$\text{Infant's dose} = \frac{\text{Age (in months)}}{\text{Average adult weight (150 lb)}} \times \text{average adult dose}$$

$$= \frac{6}{150} \times 75 \text{ mg}$$

$$= \frac{6}{\underset{2}{\cancel{150}}} \times \overset{1}{\cancel{75}} \text{ mg}$$

$$= \frac{6}{2} = 3 \text{ mg}$$

Therefore, the desired dose is 3 mg. As we know the medication is available as 1.5 mg/t, we set up the following ratio:

$$\text{Known relationship} \rightarrow \frac{1.5 \text{ mg}}{1 \text{ t}} = \frac{3 \text{ mg}}{x} \leftarrow \text{Unknown relationship}$$

$$1.5x = 3 \text{ t}$$

$$x = \frac{3 \text{ t}}{1.5}$$

$$x = 2 \text{ t}$$

Example

Child's weight: 60 lb
Average adult dose: 25 mg
How many milligrams will you administer to the child?
If the medication is available as 30 mg/T, how much fluid volume will
you give in household measures?

To Solve
Clark's rule:

$$\text{Child's dose} = \frac{\text{Weight of child in pounds}}{\text{Average adult weight (150 lb)}} \times \text{average adult dose}$$

$$= \frac{60}{150} \times 25 \text{ mg}$$

$$= \frac{6\cancel{0}}{15\cancel{0}} \times 25$$

$$= \frac{\overset{}{6}}{\underset{3}{\cancel{15}}} \times \overset{5}{\cancel{25}}$$

$$= \frac{\overset{2}{\cancel{6}}}{\underset{1}{\cancel{3}}} \times 5$$

$$= 10 \text{ mg}$$

Therefore, the desired dosage is 10 mg. We know that there is 30 mg/T
of medication and can set up the following ratio:

$$\text{Known relationship} \rightarrow \frac{30 \text{ mg}}{1 \text{ T}} = \frac{10 \text{ mg}}{x} \leftarrow \text{Unknown relationship}$$

$$30x = 10$$

$$x = \frac{10}{30}$$

$$x = \frac{1}{3} \text{ T}$$

To administer: For $\frac{1}{3}$ T you would give 1 t. You learned 3 t = 1 T. It is
always preferable to measure a full item than to approx-
imate a part of one, as it allows for greater accuracy. Because 3 t = 1 T, you would give 1 t ($= \frac{1}{3}$ T) to this child.

Example

Child's age: 6 years
Average adult dose: 36 mg
How many milligrams should be given?
If the medication is available as 4 mg per 5 cc, how much will you give in household measure?

To Solve
Young's rule:

$$\text{Child's dose} = \frac{\text{Age of child (in years)}}{\text{Age of child (in years)} + 12} \times \text{average adult dose}$$

$$= \frac{6}{6 + 12} \times 36 \text{ mg}$$

$$= \frac{6}{18} \times 36$$

$$= \frac{6}{\overset{}{\underset{1}{18}}} \times \overset{2}{36}$$

$$= 12 \text{ mg}$$

The desired dose is 12 mg and the medication available is 4 mg per 5 cc. We therefore construct the following proportion:

$$\text{Known relationship} \rightarrow \frac{4 \text{ mg}}{5 \text{ cc}} = \frac{12 \text{ mg}}{x} \leftarrow \text{Unknown relationship}$$

$$4x = 12 \times 5$$

$$x = 60 \div 4$$

$$x = 15 \text{ cc} \quad (\text{or } 1 \text{ T})$$

► When you feel that you understand this material, complete Activity Sheet 3.

Activity Sheet 3

Calculate questions 1 through 15 using either Freid's rule, Clark's rule or Young's rule.

1. If adult dosage of a drug is 100 mg/day, what would be the dosage for a child weighing 75 lb?

2. (a) The adult dosage of a drug is 400,000 to 600,000 U/day Using the maximum dosage, calculate the dose for a child weighing 60 lb.
   (b) If the medication is available as 48,000 U/cc, state how you would give it in household measure (5 cc = 1 t, 15 cc = 1 T, 30 cc = 1 oz).

3. The recommended average adult dosage of a medicine is 300 mg/day. Calculate the amount of medication per dose for an infant 10 months old.

4. (a) The adult dose of a drug is 30 mg. What is the dose for a 3-year-old child?
   (b) If the medication comes as 18 mg per 15 cc, how will this mother give this dosage in household measures?

5. The average adult dose of a drug is 1 g. What is the dose for a 4-year-old child?

6. (a) The average adult dose of a drug is 100 mg. What is the dose for a 6-month-old infant?
   (b) If the medication comes as 4 mg per 5 cc, how will you give this in household measure?

7. (a) The average adult dose is 0.6 g. What is the dosage for a 5-month-old infant?
   (b) The medication is available as 40 mg/oz. How will you give this dose in household measure?

8. A 2-month-old baby weighs 9 lb. How much medicine should be given, if the average adult dose is 750 mg?

9. An 8-year-old child needs medicine. The average adult dose is 0.4 g. How many milligrams should be given?

10. A 15-month-old infant must be given a medicine. The average adult dose is 860 mg. How much should the baby be given?

11. The average adult dose is 450 mg. The baby is 10 months old. How much medicine should be given?

12. (a) A 1-month-old infant must receive a medication. The average adult dose is 150 mg. How much should be given in milligrams?
    (b) If the medication is available as 0.5 mg per 5 cc, how much will you administer in household measure?

13. A child is 6 years old. The average adult dose is 750 mg. The medication is available as 0.125 g/T.
    (a) How many milligrams should the child receive?
    (b) How much fluid volume in household measures will you give?

14. A child weighs 25 lb. The average adult dose is 0.6 g. The medicine to give this drug is available as 50 mg per 5 cc.
    (a) How many milligrams should be given to this child?
    (b) How much fluid volume would you give in household measure?

15. An infant is 12 months old. The average adult dose is 1 g. The medication is available as 20 mg/t.
    (a) How much in grams will this infant receive?
    (b) How much in milligrams will this infant receive?
    (c) How much will you administer in household measures?

▶ Compare your answers with those at the end of this chapter. If you have answered all questions correctly, continue to the next section of text. Otherwise, review the previous text and correct your mistakes before proceeding.

INTRAVENOUS MEDICATION ADMINISTRATION

Although the administration of intravenous medications is covered in chapters 8 and 9, and the methodology you will apply here is the same, it is useful to practice with pediatric doses. Remember that pediatric doses are often very small, leaving little room for error.

Before attempting Activity Sheets 4 through 6, reread chapters 8 and 9, concentrating on the example problems calculating the flow rates for IV boluses/intermittent IV medications (piggyback bolus) and continuous medicated solutions (both for a certain amount of medication per minute and also per hour).

▶ If you did not previously complete chapters 8 and 9, you should study them before attempting Activity Sheets 4 through 6.

Activity Sheet 4

CALCULATING FLOW RATES FOR INTERMITTENT INTRAVENOUS MEDICATIONS (PIGGYBACK BOLUS)

For questions 1 through 6, answer the following:
  (a) Does the prescribed dosage level appear safe?
  (b) What flow rate should be used to administer the prescribed dose?

1. Administration set equivalency: 60 gtt = 1 cc
    Child's weight: 30 kg
    Recommended dosage:
        50–200 mg/kg per 24 hours in divided doses
    Prescribed dose: 500 mg in 25 cc D5W every 4 hours
    Administration time: 20 minutes

2. Administration set equivalency: 15 gtt = 1 cc
    Child's weight: 25 kg
    Recommended dose: 75 mg/kg every 4 hours
    Prescribed dose: 1875 mg in 50 cc NS
    Administration time: 30 minutes

3. Administration set equivalency: 60 gtt = 1 cc
    Child's weight: 40 kg
    Recommended dosage:
        1.7–3.5 mg/kg per 24 hours in four to six divided doses
    Prescribed dose: 35 mg in 60 cc D5W every 6 hours
    Administration time: 45 minutes

4. Administration set equivalency: 15 gtt = 1 cc
    Child's weight: 11 lb
    Recommended dosage: 100 mg/kg
    Prescribed dose: 400 mg in 20 cc D5W
    Administration time: 15 minutes

5. Administration set equivalency: 10 gtt = 1 cc
   Child's weight: 88 lb
   Recommended dosage: 200–350 mg/kg/day in divided doses
   Prescribed dose: 2 g in 150 cc NS every 6 hours
   Administration time: 90 minutes

6. Administration set equivalency: 20 gtt = 1 cc
   Child's size: 1.3 m²
   Recommended dosage: 250 mg/m² every 8 hours
   Prescribed dose: 325 mg in 75 cc D5W
   Administration time: 1 hour

▶   Compare your answers with those at the end of this chapter. If you have answered all
    questions correctly, continue to Activity Sheet 5. Otherwise, review the text and examples
    in chapters 8 and 9 and correct your mistakes on this activity sheet before proceeding.

Activity Sheet 5

CALCULATING FLOW RATES FOR CONTINUOUS MEDICATED SOLUTIONS PRESCRIBED DOSE PER MINUTE

For questions 1 through 5, calculate the flow rate to administer the prescribed dose. The administration set equivalency is 60 gtt = 1 cc.

1. Medicated solution: 6 g per 100 cc D5W
   Recommended dosage: no greater than 60 mg/min
   Prescribed dose: 45 mg/min

2. Medicated solution: 10 g per 200 cc D5W
   Recommended dosage: no greater than 50 mg/min
   Prescribed dose: 12.5 mg/min

3. Medicated solution: 0.8 g per 200 cc
   Recommended dosage: 20–40 μg/kg/min
   Child's weight: 40 kg
   Prescribed dose: 25 μg/kg/min

4. Medicated solution: 2.1 g per 200 cc
   Recommended dosage: 20–80 μg/kg/min
   Child's weight: 30 kg
   Prescribed dose: 70 μg/kg/min

5. Medicated solution: 350 mg per 500 cc
   Recommended dosage: 20–40 mcg/kg/min
   Child's weight: 35 kg
   Prescribed dose: 20 mcg/kg/min

▶ Compare your answers with those at the end of this chapter. If you have answered all questions correctly, continue to Activity Sheet 6. Otherwise, review the text and examples in chapters 8 and 9 and correct your mistakes on this activity sheet before continuing.

Activity Sheet 6

CALCULATING FLOW RATES FOR CONTINUOUS MEDICATED SOLUTIONS PRESCRIBED DOSE PER HOUR

For the following problems calculate:
- (a) the amount of medication the child should receive per hour,
- (b) the flow rate (gtt/min) necessary to administer that amount, and
- (c) the amount of cc/hr that should be administered to provide that dose.

The administration set equivalency is 60 gtt = 1 cc.

1. Medicated solution: 500 mg per 500 cc
   Child's weight: 40 kg
   Prescribed dose: 1.0 mg/kg/hr

2. Medicated solution: 400 mg per 500 cc
   Child's weight: 30 kg
   Prescribed dose: 1.2 mg/kg/hr

3. Medicated solution: 250 mg per 250 cc
   Child's weight: 20 kg
   Prescribed dose: 0.8 mg/kg/hr

4. Medicated solution: 500 mg per 500 cc
   Child's weight: 10 kg
   Prescribed dose: 1.1 mg/kg/hr

5. Medicated solution: 200 mg per 250 cc
   Child's weight: 20 kg
   Prescribed dose: 0.4 mg/kg/hr

▶ Compare your answers with those at the end of this chapter. If you have answered all questions correctly, take the posttest. Otherwise, review the text and examples in chapters 8 and 9 and correct your mistakes on this activity sheet before proceeding.

Posttest

1. Why must you be able to calculate infant's and children's dosages accurately and be able to recognize unusual dosage amounts?

2. Child's weight: 66 lb
   Recommended dose: 0.01 mg/kg
   Medication available: 0.25 mg/cc
   The child's dose should be _____ mg.
   You will give therefore _____ cc.

3. Child's weight: 55 lb
   Recommended dose: 60 µg/kg
   Medication available: 1 mg/cc
   The child's dose should be _____ µg.
   You will give therefore _____ cc.

4. Child's weight: 88 lb
   Recommended dose: 100 U/kg
   Medication available: 5000 U/cc
   The child's dose should be _____ U.
   You will give therefore _____ cc.

5. Child's weight: 30 kg
   Recommended dose: 0.1 mg/lb
   Medication available: 3 mg/cc
   The child's dose should be _____ mg.
   You will give therefore _____ cc.

6. Child's weight: 22 lb
   Recommended dose: 20 µg/kg
   Medication available: 2 mg/cc
   The child should receive _____ µg.
   You will give therefore _____ cc.

7. Child's body surface: 0.7 m^2
   Prescribed dose: 750 mg/m^2/day
   The child should receive _____ mg/day.

TPO   IPO
2

8. Child's body surface: 1.1 m^2
   Prescribed dose: 250 mg/m^2 every 8 hours
   The child should receive _____ mg every 8 hours.

2

9. Body surface: 1.0 m^2
   Average adult dose: 1000 mcg
   The child should receive _____ mcg.

2

10. Body surface: 0.6 m^2
    Average adult dose: 500 mg
    The child should receive _____ mg.

3,8

11. (a) The baby is 2 months old. The average adult dose is 0.75 g. You
         will administer _____ mg.
    (b) The medication available is 5 mg per 5 cc. How much will you
         administer in household measure?

3,8

12. (a) A child weighs 25 lb. The average adult dose is 0.12 g. You will
         administer _____ mg.
    (b) If the medication is available as 40 mg/oz, how much will you
         give in household measure?

3,8

13. (a) A child is 2 years old. The average adult dose is 0.42 g. You will
         administer _____ mg.
    (b) If the medication is available as 360 mg/oz, how much will you
         give in household measure?

4

14. Administration set equivalency: 15 gtt = 1 cc
    Child's weight: 77 lb
    Recommended dose: 1.7–3.5 mg/kg per 24 hours in four to six di-
                      vided doses
    Prescribed dose: 30 mg in 50 D5W every 4 hours
    Administration time: 30 minutes
    Does the prescribed dose appear to be a safe dosage level?
    What flow rate should be used to administer this dose?

4

15. Administration set equivalency: 60 gtt = 1 cc
    Child's body surface: 0.5 m^2
    Recommended dose: 250 mg/m^2 every 8 hours
    Prescribed dose: 125 mg in 60 cc NS every 8 hours
    Administration time: 45 minutes
    Does this prescribed dose appear accurate/safe?
    What flow rate should be used to administer this prescribed dose?

TPO   IPO

For questions 16 through 21, the administration set equivalency is 60 gtt = 1 cc.

5

16. Medicated solution: 5 g per 100 cc NS
Recommended dosage: no faster than 50 mg/min
Prescribed dose: 30 mg/min
What flow rate should be used to administer the prescribed dose?

5

17. Medicated solution: 12 g per 200 cc D5W
Recommended dosage: no greater than 60 mg/min
Prescribed dose: 37 mg/min
What flow rate should be used to administer this prescribed dose?

5

18. Medicated solution: 0.4 g per 200 cc
Recommended dosage: 20–40 µg/kg/min
Child's weight: 66 lb
Prescribed dose: 20 µg/kg/min
What flow rate should be used to administer the prescribed dose?

5

19. Medicated solution: 1.25 g per 1000 cc
Recommended dosage: 20–40 mcg/kg/min
Child's weight: 25 kg
Prescribed dose: 25 mcg/kg/min
What flow rate should be used to administer the prescribed dose?

6

20. Medicated solution: 250 mg per 250 cc
Child's weight: 40 kg
Prescribed dosage: 0.9 mg/kg/hr
How much medication per hour should this child receive?
What flow rate should be used to administer this?
How many cc/hr will this child receive?

6

21. Medicated solution: 200 mg per 250 cc
Child's weight: 32 kg
Prescribed dose: 0.5 mg/kg/hr
How much medication per hour will this child receive?
What flow rate should be used to administer this?
How many cc/hr will this child receive?

▶   Compare your answers with those at the end of the chapter. If you have answered all questions correctly, go on to chapter 11. Otherwise, note the objective next to the problems you answered incorrectly, review the text relative to this, and correct your mistakes. Then take the pretest of this chapter as a second posttest before proceeding.

Answers for Chapter 10

PRETEST

1. To ensure the administration of safe dosages
2. 0.25, 1
3. 1200, 1.2
4. 3000, 0.6   5. 9.9, 3.3   6. 800, 0.4
7. 675   8. 300   9. 462
10. 332   11. (a) 3   (b) 1 T
12. (a) 80   (b) 2   13. (a) 60   (b) 1   14. Yes; 25 gtt/min
15. Yes; 100 gtt/min   16. 45 gtt/min
17. 15 gtt/min   18. 36 gtt/min
19. 60 gtt/min   20. 45 mg, 45 gtt/min, 45
21. 20 mg, 25 gtt/min, 25

ACTIVITY SHEET 1

1. (a) 25 mg per 24 hours in two divided doses, that is, 12.5 mg twice a day
   (b) $\frac{1}{2}$ tablet twice a day
2. (a) 13.5 mg   (b) 4.5 mL
3. (a) 4.5 mg   (b) 1.5 mL
4. (a) 1400 mcg   (b) 1.4 cc
5. (a) 0.7 mg   (b) 2.8 cc   (*Note:* 77 lb = 35 kg)
6. (a) 3200 U   (b) 3.2 cc
7. (a), (b) = 3.2 cc
8. (a) 800 μg   (b) 0.4 cc
9. (a) 4500 U   (b) 0.9 cc
10. (a), (b) 0.4 cc

ACTIVITY SHEET 2

1. 600 mg/day
2. 260 mg
3. 187.5 mg every 8 hours
4. 325 mg
5. 275 mg three times daily
6. 289 mg
7. 975 mg per 24 hours
8. 90 mg

ACTIVITY SHEET 3

1. 50 mg
2. (a) 240, 000 U   (b) 1 t
3. 20 mg
4. (a) 6 mg   (b) 1 t
5. 0.25 g
6. (a) 4 mg   (b) 1 t
7. (a) 20 mg   (b) 1 T
8. 10 mg
9. 160 mg
10. 86 mg
11. 30 mg
12. (a) 1 mg   (b) 2 t
13. (a) 250   (b) 2 T (1 oz)
14. (a) 100   (b) 2 t
15. (a) 0.08   (b) 80   (c) 1 t + 1 T

ACTIVITY SHEET 4

1. (a) Yes   (b) 75 gtt/min   2. (a) Yes   (b) 25 gtt/min
3. (a) Yes   (b) 80 gtt/min   4. (a) Yes   (b) 20 gtt/min
5. (a) Yes   (b) 16–17 gtt/min   6. (a) Yes   (b) 25 gtt/min

ACTIVITY SHEET 5

1. 45 gtt/min   2. 15 gtt/min   3. 15 gtt/min
4. 12 gtt/min   5. 60 gtt/min

ACTIVITY SHEET 6

1. (a) 40 mg/hr   (b) 40 gtt/min   (c) 40 cc/hr
2. (a) 36 mg/hr   (b) 45 gtt/min   (c) 45 cc/hr
3. (a) 16 mg/hr   (b) 16 gtt/min   (c) 16 cc/hr
4. (a) 11 mg/hr   (b) 11 gtt/min   (c) 11 cc/hr
5. (a)   8 mg/hr   (b) 10 gtt/min   (c) 10 cc/hr

POSTTEST

1. To ensure the administration of safe dosages
2. 0.3, 1.2
3. 1500, 1.5
4. 4000, 0.8
5. 6.6, 2.2
6. 200, 0.1
7. 525
8. 275
9. 578
10. 173
11. (a) 10   (b) 2 t
12. (a) 20   (b) 1 T
13. (a) 60   (b) 1 t
14. No, 25 gtt/min
15. Yes, 80 gtt/min
16. 36 gtt/min
17. 37 gtt/min
18. 18 gtt/min
19. 30 gtt/min
20. 36 mg/hr, 36 gtt/min, 36 cc/hr
21. 16 mg/hr, 20 gtt/min, 20 cc/hr

11 | *Preparation of Solutions*

TERMINAL PERFORMANCE OBJECTIVES

1. Given a prescribed concentration strength of medication, the reader is able to state or compute the amount of active ingredient (solute) to be used and the amount of fluid volume (solvent/diluent) to be used in order to obtain this concentration strength.
2. Given a prescribed amount of solution to administer of a specified percentage concentration, the reader is able to calculate the amount of solute and solvent to use to prepare this.

INTERMEDIATE PERFORMANCE OBJECTIVES

After studying the text, the reader is able to:

1. List the component parts of a solution.
2. Compare and contrast the difference in measuring the total volume of a solution when the active ingredient is dry as opposed to when it is liquid.
3. State the basis for determining the amount of total fluid volume to prepare when it is not prescribed.
4. Compute the total amount of medication needed for a specific fluid volume and concentration strength.
5. Compute the amount of solute necessary for a prescribed solution.

6. State or calculate the amount of solvent necessary for a prescribed solution.

7. Calculate the amount of solute and solvent necessary to prepare a specified solution measured in percent.

▶   If you feel confident that you possess these skills, take the pretest. Otherwise, begin to study the material in this chapter.

Pretest

For the questions 1 through 5, calculate (a) the amount of medication to be contained in the entire preparation, (b) the volume or amount of solute, and (c) the volume of solvent.

1   1–6   1. Prescribed solution: 3:1 concentration (3 mg/cc)
Medication available: 0.3 g per 10 cc
Decided total solution amount: 300 cc

1   1–6   2. Prescribed solution: 25:1 concentration (25 U/cc)
Medication available: 500 U per 10 cc
Decided total solution amount: 500 cc

1   1–6   3. Prescribed solution: 5:1 concentration (5 mcg/cc)
Medication available: 0.5 mg per 5 cc
Decided total solution amount: 1000 cc

1   1–6   4. Prescribed solution: 4:1 concentration (4 mg/cc)
Medication available: 0.125 g per tablet (or powdered form)
Decided total solution amount: 250 cc

1   1–6   5. Prescribed solution: 10:1 concentration (10 mcg/cc)
Medication available: 0.25 mg per tablet (or powdered form)
Decided total solution amount: 200 cc

For questions 6 through 11, calculate the amount of (a) solute and (b) solvent necessary.

1   1–3,5,6   6. Prescribed medicated solution: 1.75 g in 1000 cc
Medication available: 500 mg per 10 cc

1   1–3,5,6   7. Prescribed medicated solution: 3 mg per 500 cc
Medication available: 100 mcg per 5 cc

1   1–3,5,6   8. Prescribed medicated solution: 55,000 U per 500 cc
Medication available: 1000 U/cc

TPO	IPO
1	1–3,5,6
1	1–3,5,6
1	1–3,5,6
2	1,2,7
2	1,2,7
2	1,2,7
2	1,2,7
2	1,2,7
2	1,2,7

9. Prescribed medicated solution: 125 mg per 300 cc
   Medication available: 25 mg per tablet (or powdered form)

10. Prescribed medicated solution: 0.05 mg per 2 cc
    Medication available: 0.1 mg per vial (powdered form)

11. Prescribed medicated solution: 250 mg/cc
    Medication available: 2 g per vial (powdered form)

For questions 12 through 17, calculate the amount of (a) solute and (b) solvent necessary to prepare the solution.

12. Prescribed solution: 250 cc of a 40% solution
    Preparation available (solute): 100% solution

13. Prescribed solution: 1000 cc of a 0.5% solution
    Preparation available (solute): 5% solution

14. Prescribed solution: 500 cc of a 9% solution
    Preparation available (solute): 60% solution

15. Prescribed solution: 1000 cc of a 0.25% solution
    Solute: dry form

16. Prescribed solution: 500 cc of a 4.5% solution
    Solute: dry form

17. Prescribed solution: 250 cc of a 30% solution
    Solute: dry form

▶ Compare your answers with those at the end of this chapter. If you have answered all questions correctly, proceed to Chapter 12. Otherwise, begin to study the material in this chapter.

CONCENTRATION OF MEDICATED SOLUTIONS

There may be situations where you will have to prepare a solution in a specified concentration. There are, of course, two parts to every solution—the solute, which is the active ingredient, and the solvent, which is the substance that is used as the diluting agent. The solute is commonly measured in grams, milligrams, micrograms, units, milliequivalents, and so on. The solvent corresponds to the vehicle. In preparing solutions we are dealing, of course, with vehicles of liquid measures only. We will not be concerned in this chapter with the types of diluents used, because that will be prescribed by either the physician or the accompanying reference literature. What will concern us is the amount of the vehicle or diluent, for this is an important aspect of our mathematical calculations.

The total volume of a solution is the volume of the active ingredient (solute) plus the volume of the vehicle (solvent). When both of these component parts are liquids, the total volume of a solution is obtained by summing the volumes of the component parts. When the solute is a dry or powdered ingredient, however, the process is not as easy, for the solute is dispersed throughout the solvent and the total volume is not equal to the pure mathematical sum of the two. One must measure the total amount that occurs after the two component parts are mixed together.

The total fluid volume that is necessary to prepare in a situation may be prescribed, or it may be a volume that you determine. If you have to determine the volume to prepare, you must keep in mind the purpose for which the medication is intended. This will give you an idea of the fluid volume that you will need. For example, the fluid volume required for an injection is certainly less than that required for a medicated foot soak.

The remainder of this chapter presents examples of situations that you might encounter clinically. It is difficult to say how often you will be required to complete such tasks. With increasing frequency, the pharmacy is preparing medicated solutions. The guides and practice problems that follow will enable you to meet the clinical expectations that do arise.

▶   When you feel confident that you understand this material, complete Activity Sheet 1.

Activity Sheet 1

1. What are the component parts of a solution?

2. Active ingredient corresponds to which component of a solution?

3. To which component of a solution does the term vehicle correspond?

4. List five common measurements of active ingredients.

5. What comprises the total volume of a solution?

6. How would you measure the total volume of a solution when both the component parts are liquid?

7. Discuss the measurement of the total volume of a solution when the solute is in dry form.

8. If the total volume of solution necessary to prepare is not prescribed, what will be your basis for deciding how much of a volume to prepare?

▶ Compare your answers with those at the end of this chapter. If you have answered all questions correctly, continue to the text that follows. Otherwise, review the preceding text and correct your mistakes before continuing.

UNSPECIFIED VOLUME WITH LIQUID SOLUTE

Example

Prescribed solution: 4:1 concentration (4 mg/cc)
Total fluid volume: 200 cc is needed (amount decided by preparer)
Medication available: 50 mg/cc

To Solve

1. Compute the total amount of medication needed for the specified fluid volume and concentration.

    The required concentration per cubic centimeter is equal to the required concentration of the total fluid volume, that is,

$$\frac{4 \text{ mg}}{1 \text{ cc}} = \frac{x \text{ (mg)}}{200 \text{ cc}}$$

$$x = 4 \times 200$$

$$x = 800 \text{ mg}$$

2. Compute the amount of solute necessary.

    Relate the available medication to the amount of medication necessary for the entire prepared solution:

$$\frac{50 \text{ mg}}{1 \text{ cc}} = \frac{800 \text{ mg}}{x \text{ (cc)}}$$

$$50x = 800$$

$$x = 800 \div 50$$

$$x = 16 \text{ cc (of the 50 mg/cc medication)}$$

3. Calculate the amount of solvent necessary.

    The total solution volume is equal to the amount of liquid solute plus amount of solvent. Therefore,

$$\text{Solvent} = \text{Total fluid volume} - \text{volume of solute}$$

$$= 200 \text{ cc} - 16 \text{ cc}$$

$$= 184 \text{ cc}$$

Final answer: use 16 cc of the 50 mg/cc solute and add 184 cc of solvent to obtain a 4:1 concentration of 800 mg per 200 cc.

UNSPECIFIED VOLUME WITH DRY SOLUTE

Example

Prescribed solution: 10:1 concentration (10 mg/cc)
Medication available: 500 mg per tablet or powdered form
Decide on a solution amount: 250 cc

To Solve

1. Compute the amount of medication necessary for the specified concentration and fluid volume.

 The required concentration per cubic centimeter is equal to the required concentration of the total fluid volume, that is,

$$\frac{10 \text{ mg}}{1 \text{ cc}} = \frac{x \text{ (mg)}}{250 \text{ cc}}$$

$$x = 10 \times 250$$

$$x = 2500 \text{ mg}$$

2. Compute the amount of solute needed.

 Relate the available medication to the amount of medication necessary for the entire prepared solution:

$$\frac{500 \text{ mg}}{1 \text{ tablet}} = \frac{2500 \text{ mg}}{x \text{ (tablets)}}$$

$$500x = 2500$$

$$x = 2500 \div 500$$

$$x = 5 \text{ tablets}$$

3. Determine the amount of solvent.

 Dissolve the tablets in a small amount of the solvent first, and then add more solvent until you reach the desired amount—for this problem, 250 cc.

▶ When you feel confident that you understand this material, complete Activity Sheet 2.

Activity Sheet 2

For questions 1 through 8, calculate (a) the amount of medication to be contained in the entire preparation, (b) the volume of solute, and (c) the volume of solvent. (Frequently, in clinical situations you will be required to choose the total fluid volume, but for practice in determining your accuracy, a volume is assigned here.)

1. Prescribed solution: 3:1 concentration (3 mg/cc)
   Medication available: 50 mg per 2 cc
   Total fluid volume chosen: 250 cc

2. Prescribed solution: 2:1 concentration (2 mcg/cc)
   Medication available: 0.5 mg per 20 cc
   Total fluid volume chosen: 1000 cc

3. Prescribed solution: 5:1 concentration (5 mg/cc)
   Medication available: 0.5 g per 25 cc
   Total fluid volume chosen: 200 cc

4. Prescribed solution: 4:1 concentration (4 U/cc)
   Medication available: 500 U per 5 cc
   Total fluid volume chosen: 500 cc

5. Prescribed solution: 20:1 concentration (20 U/cc)
   Medication available: 500 U/cc
   Total fluid volume chosen: 1000 cc

6. Prescribed solution: 4:1 concentration (4 mg/cc)
   Medication available: 0.5 g per tablet
   Total fluid volume chosen: 1000 cc

7. Prescribed solution: 3:1 concentration (3 mcg/cc)
   Medication available: 0.4 mg per tablet
   Total fluid volume chosen: 400 cc

8. Prescribed solution: 15:1 concentration (15 U/cc)
   Medication available: 1000 U per tablet
   Total fluid volume chosen: 500 cc

▶   Compare your answers with those at the end of this chapter. If you have answered all questions correctly, continue to the text that follows. Otherwise, review the previous text and correct your mistakes before proceeding.

SPECIFIED VOLUME WITH LIQUID SOLUTE

Example

Prescribed medicated solution: 100 mg per 250 cc
Available medication: 50 mg per 5 cc
Amount of solute to use: _____
Amount of solvent to use: _____

To Solve

1. Calculate the amount of medication to use (solute).
   Relate the available medication to the amount of medication necessary for the entire prepared solution:

$$\frac{50 \text{ mg}}{5 \text{ cc}} = \frac{100 \text{ mg}}{x \text{ (cc)}}$$

$$50x = 5 \times 100$$

$$50x = 500$$

$$x = 500 \div 50$$

$$x = 10 \text{ cc (of the medication containing 50 mg per 5 cc)}$$

2. Calculate the amount of solvent.

$$\text{Solvent} = \text{Total volume} - \text{amount of liquid solute}$$

$$= 250 \text{ cc} - 10 \text{ cc}$$

$$= 240 \text{ cc}$$

SPECIFIED VOLUME WITH DRY SOLUTE

Example

Prescribed medicated solution: 125 mg per 250 cc
Medication available: 25 mg per tablet
Amount of solute to use: _____
Amount of solvent to use: _____

To Solve

1. Calculate the amount of solute needed.
   Relate the medication available to the amount of medication necessary for the entire prepared solution:

$$\frac{25 \text{ mg}}{1 \text{ tablet}} = \frac{125 \text{ mg}}{x \text{ (tablet)}}$$

$$25x = 125$$

$$x = 125 \div 25$$

$$x = 5 \text{ tablets}$$

2. Determine the amount of solute to use.
   In an appropriate container dissolve the dry solute and then add sufficient fluid to equal the needed prescribed volume.

Example

Prescribed medicated solution: 25 mg/cc
Medication available: 50 mg per vial (powdered form)
Amount of solute to use: _____
Amount of solvent to use: _____

To Solve

1. Calculate the amount of solute needed.

   Relate the medication available to the amount of medication necessary for the entire prepared solution:

   $$\frac{50 \text{ mg}}{1 \text{ vial}} = \frac{25 \text{ mg}}{x \text{ (vial)}}$$

   $$50x = 25$$

   $$x = 25 \div 50$$

   $$x = \frac{1}{2} \text{ vial}$$

2. Determine the amount of solute to use.

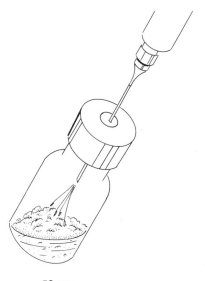

50 mg

There are two doses in this vial. Therefore, a total volume of 2 cc is required in order to give these two doses. To prepare the solution add a small amount of liquid, say 1 cc, to make the powder a fluid, and then add liquid until the total volume equals 2 cc. This gives you 50 mg per 2 cc or 25 mg/cc. Be sure to label the vial as to the concentration and date and time of preparation and expiration, and sign your initials.

▶   When you feel confident that you understand this material, complete Activity Sheet 3.

Activity Sheet 3

For the following problems calculate the amount of (a) solute and (b) solvent necessary for the given facts.

1. Prescribed medicated solution: 120 mg per 200 cc
   Available medication: 40 mg per 10 cc

2. Prescribed medicated solution: 50 mEq per 200 cc
   Available medication: 20 mEq per 20 cc

3. Prescribed medicated solution: 45,000 U per 1000 cc
   Available medication: 1000 U/cc

4. Prescribed medicated solution: 4 mg per 500 cc
   Available medication: 200 mcg per 5 cc

5. Prescribed medicated solution: 1.5 g per 750 L
   Available medication: 250 mg per 10 cc

6. Prescribed medication solution: 50 mg per 200 cc
   Available medication: 12.5 mg per tablet

7. Prescribed medicated solution: 50 mg/cc
   Available medication: 100 mg/powder in vial

8. Prescribed medicated solution: 0.375 g per 500 cc
   Available medication: 125 mg per tablet

9. Prescribed medicated solution: 15 mg per 0.5 cc
   Available medication: 45 mg in a vial (powdered form)

10. Prescribed medicated solution: 0.125 mcg per 2 cc
    Available medication: 0.25 mcg of powder in a vial

▶ Compare your answers with those at the end of this chapter. If you have answered all questions correctly, continue to the text that follows. Otherwise, review the preceding text and correct your mistakes before proceeding.

PREPARING PERCENTAGE SOLUTIONS

On occasion you may need to prepare a solution whose concentration is measured as a percent, for example, 50%, 3%, or 0.9%. This percent refers to the concentration of the active ingredient. If you do not know the total volume of solution but only the concentration strength, then you should base your calculations on a 100 cc quantity. For example, if you are told that you have available a 50% stock solution, this means that 50 cc of every 100 cc is the active ingredient (solute) and 50 cc is the diluent (solvent).

Although we have used the proportion method throughout most of this text, this is one of the few instances in which the formula method of drug calculation, explained in chapter 4, is a better method to employ. The examples that follow will illustrate the ease with which these problems can be solved.

Example

Prescribed solution: 500 cc of a 40% solution concentration
Preparation available: 100%
In the prescribed solution there is _____ cc solute and _____ cc solvent.

To Solve

1. Compute the amount of solute (active ingredient) for the prescribed solution.

$$\text{Amount of solute} = \frac{\text{Prescribed concentration}}{\text{Preparation available}} \times \begin{array}{c}\text{total}\\\text{quantity}\\\text{desired}\end{array}$$

$$= \frac{40\%}{100\%} \times 500 \text{ cc}$$

$$= 200 \text{ cc}$$

2. Calculate the amount of solvent necessary for the prescribed solution.

The total fluid volume is equal to the volume of solute plus the volume of solvent; therefore,

$$\text{Volume of solvent} = \text{Total fluid volume} - \text{volume of solute}$$

$$= 500 \text{ cc} - 200 \text{ cc}$$

$$= 300 \text{ cc}$$

Example

Prescribed solution: 1000 mL of a 50% solution
Preparation available: 80% stock solution
In the prescribed solution there is _____ mL of solute and _____ mL of solvent.

To Solve

1. Calculate the volume of solute. (Use the same formula as in the previous example.)

$$\text{Amount of solute} = \frac{50\%}{80\%} \times 1000 \text{ mL}$$

$$= 625 \text{ mL}$$

2. Calculate the amount of solvent.

$$\text{Amount of solvent} = \text{Total fluid volume} - \text{volume of solute}$$

$$= 1000 \text{ mL} - 625 \text{ mL}$$

$$= 375 \text{ mL}$$

To prepare a solution for the situation when the solute is in dry form, one must consider that the amount of solute or active ingredient necessary depends directly on the relationship between the prescribed percent of the solution and the volume of solution needed. This is very easy to calculate, as the following example will illustrate.

Example

Prescribed solution: 500 cc of a 5% solution
For the prescribed amount and concentration of solution _____ g of solute and _____ cc of solvent are necessary.

To Solve

1. Calculate the amount of solute.

$$\text{Amount of solute} = \text{Prescribed percent} \times \text{total fluid volume}$$

$$= 5\% \times 500 \text{ cc}$$

$$= 0.05 \times 500 = 25 \text{ g}$$

2. Determine the amount of solvent.
    Place the solute (25 g) in an appropriate container and add the solvent until you reach the prescribed total volume, 500 cc.

▶   When you feel confident that you understand this material, complete Activity Sheet 4.

Activity Sheet 4

For questions 1 through 8, calculate the amount of (a) liquid solute and (b) solvent necessary to prepare the solutions based on the given facts.

1. Prescribed solution: 250 cc of a 2% solution
   Preparation available: 50% of stock solution

2. Prescribed solution: 500 cc of a 0.9% solution
   Preparation available: 10% solution

3. Prescribed solution: 100 cc of a 10% solution
   Preparation available: 100% solution

4. Prescribed solution: 1000 cc of a 25% solution
   Preparation available: 50% solution

5. Prescribed solution: 750 cc of a 25% solution
   Preparation available: 75% solution

6. Prescribed solution: 500 cc of an 0.8% solution
   Preparation available: 100% solution

7. Prescribed solution: 200 cc of a 5% solution
   Preparation available: 25% solution

8. Prescribed solution: 50 cc of a 2.5% solution
   Preparation available: 100% solution

For questions 9 through 16, calculate the amount of (a) dry solute and (b) solvent necessary for the prescribed solution.

9. Prescribed solution: 1000 cc of a 10% solution

10. Prescribed solution: 1000 cc of a 0.9% solution

11. Prescribed solution: 500 cc of a 35% solution

12. Prescribed solution: 250 cc of an 8% solution

13. Prescribed solution: 300 cc of a 2.5% solution

14. Prescribed solution: 1000 cc of a 0.45% solution

15. Prescribed solution: 750 cc of a 1% solution

16. Prescribed solution: 200 cc of a 75% solution

▶ Compare your answers with those at the end of this chapter. If you have answered all questions correctly, take the posttest. Otherwise, review the previous text and correct your mistakes before taking the posttest.

Posttest

For questions 1 through 5, calculate (a) the amount of medication to be contained in the entire preparation, (b) the volume of solute, and (c) the volume of solvent.

1. Prescribed solution: 3:1 concentration (3 mg/cc)
   Medication available: 0.5 g per 25 cc
   Decided total solution amount: 500 cc

2. Prescribed solution: 25:1 concentration (25 U/cc)
   Medication available: 500 U per 10 cc
   Decided total solution amount: 1000 cc

3. Prescribed solution: 5:1 concentration (5 mcg/cc)
   Medication available: 0.25 mg per 2 cc
   Decided total solution amount: 500 cc

4. Prescribed solution: 4:1 concentration (4 mg/cc)
   Medication available: 0.8 g per tablet
   Decided total solution amount: 400 cc

5. Prescribed solution: 10:1 concentration (10 mcg/cc)
   Medication available: 1 mg per tablet
   Decided total solution amount: 250 cc

For questions 6 through 11, calculate the amount of (a) solute and (b) solvent.

6. Prescribed medicated solution: 1.25 g per 250 cc
   Medication available: 250 mg per 5 cc

7. Prescribed medicated solution: 2 mg per 1000 cc
   Medication available: 100 mcg per 10 cc

8. Prescribed medicated solution: 25,000 U per 500 cc
   Medication available: 1000 U/cc

TPO	IPO
1	1–3,5,6
1	1–3,5,6
1	1–3,5,6
2	1,2,7
2	1,2,7
2	1,2,7
2	1,2,7
2	1,2,7
2	1,2,7

9. Prescribed medicated solution: 90 mg per 200 cc
Medication available: 30 mg per tablet

10. Prescribed medicated solution: 0.125 mg/cc
Medication available: 0.5 mg per vial

11. Prescribed medicated solution: 200 mg per 2 cc
Medication available: 1 g per vial

For questions 12 through 17, calculate the amount of (a) solute and (b) solvent.

12. Prescribed solution: 500 cc of a 25% solution
Preparation available: solute liquid, 100% solution

13. Prescribed solution: 1000 cc of a 0.9% solution
Preparation available: solute liquid, 100% solution

14. Prescribed solution: 250 cc of a 10% solution
Preparation available: solute liquid, 50% solution

15. Prescribed solution: 1000 cc of a 0.35% solution
Solute is in dry form.

16. Prescribed solution: 500 cc of a 2.5% solution
Solute is in dry form.

17. Prescribed solution: 250 cc of a 20% solution
Solute is in dry form.

▶ Compare your answers with those at the end of this chapter. If you have answered all questions correctly, proceed to chapter 12. Otherwise, note the number next to your incorrect test item, return to the relevant text, review it, and practice the appropriate items on the activity sheets. Then correct your mistakes on this test and take the pretest of this chapter as a second posttest before continuing.

Answers for Chapter 11

1. (a) 900 mg   (b) 30 cc   (c) 270 cc
2. (a) 12,500 U   (b) 250 cc   (c) 250 cc
3. (a) 5000 mcg   (b) 50 cc   (c) 950 cc
4. (a) 1000 mg   (b) 8 tablets
   (c) Liquefy the tablets and add fluid to 250 cc.
5. (a) 2000 mcg   (b) 8 tablets
   (c) Liquefy the tablets and add fluid to 200 cc.
6. (a) 35 cc   (b) 965 cc
7. (a) 150 cc   (b) 350 cc
8. (a) 55 cc   (b) 445 cc
9. (a) 5 tablets
   (b) Liquefy the tablets and add fluid to 300 cc.
10. (a) $\frac{1}{2}$ vial
    (b) Liquefy the powder and add fluid to 4 cc; two doses of 0.05 mg/ 2 cc.
11. (a) $\frac{1}{8}$ vial
    (b) Liquefy the powder and add fluid to 8 cc; eight doses of 250 mg/ cc.
12. (a) 100 cc   (b) 150 cc
13. (a) 100 cc   (b) 900 cc
14. (a) 75 cc   (b) 425 cc
15. (a) 2.5 g   (b) Fluid to 1000 cc
16. (a) 22.5 g   (b) Fluid to 500 cc
17. (a) 75 g   (b) Fluid to 250 cc

ACTIVITY SHEET 1

1. Solute and solvent
2. Solute
3. Solvent
4. Grams, milligrams, micrograms, units, milliequivalents
5. The volume of solute plus the volume of solvent
6. Add the two volumes.
7. You must measure the volume after the solute and solvent are mixed.
8. The intended purpose of the solution

ACTIVITY SHEET 2

1. (a) 750 mg   (b) 30 cc   (c) 220 cc
2. (a) 2000 mcg   (b) 80 cc   (c) 920 cc
3. (a) 1000 mg   (b) 50 cc   (c) 150 cc
4. (a) 2000 U   (b) 20 cc   (c) 480 cc
5. (a) 20,000 U   (b) 40 cc   (c) 960 cc
6. (a) 4000 mg   (b) 8 tablets
   (c) Liquefy the tablets and add solution to 1000 cc.
7. (a) 1200 mcg   (b) 3 tablets
   (c) Liquefy the tablets and add solution to 400 cc.
8. (a) 7500 U   (b) 7.5 tablets
   (c) Liquefy the tablets and add solution to 500 cc.

ACTIVITY SHEET 3

1. (a) 30 cc   (b) 170 cc
2. (a) 50 cc   (b) 150 cc
3. (a) 45 cc   (b) 955 cc
4. (a) 100 cc   (b) 400 cc
5. (a) 60 cc   (b) 690 cc
6. (a) 4 tablets   (b) Liquefy the tablets and add solution to 200 cc.

7. (a) $\frac{1}{2}$ vial

   (b) Liquefy the powder and add fluid up to 2 cc; you will have two doses of 50 mg/cc.

8. (a) 3 tablets

   (b) Liquefy the tablets and add fluid up to 500 cc.

9. (a) $\frac{1}{3}$ vial

   (b) Liquefy the powder and add fluid to a 1.5 cc total; you will have three doses of 15 mg/0.5 cc.

10. (a) $\frac{1}{2}$ vial

    (b) Liquefy the powder and add fluid to a volume of 4 cc; you will have two doses of 0.125 mcg per 2 cc.

ACTIVITY SHEET 4

1. (a) 10 cc   (b) 240 cc
2. (a) 45 cc   (b) 455 cc
3. (a) 10 cc   (b) 90 cc
4. (a) 500 cc   (b) 500 cc
5. (a) 250 cc   (b) 500 cc
6. (a) 4 cc   (b) 496 cc
7. (a) 40 cc   (b) 160 cc
8. (a) $1\frac{1}{4}$ (1.25) cc   (b) $48\frac{3}{4}$ (48.75) cc
9. (a) 100 g   (b) Fluid to 1000 cc
10. (a) 9 g   (b) Fluid to 1000 cc
11. (a) 175 g   (b) Fluid to 500 cc
12. (a) 20 g   (b) Fluid to 250 cc
13. (a) 7.5 g   (b) Fluid to 300 cc
14. (a) 4.5 g   (b) Fluid to 1000 cc
15. (a) 7.5 g   (b) Fluid to 750 cc
16. (a) 150 g   (b) Fluid to 200 cc

POSTTEST

1. (a) 1500 mg   (b) 75 cc   (c) 425 cc
2. (a) 25,000 U   (b) 500 cc   (c) 500 cc
3. (a) 2500 mcg   (b) 20 cc   (c) 480 cc
4. (a) 1600 mg   (b) 2 tablets
   (c) Liquefy the tablets and add fluid to 400 cc.
5. (a) 2500 mcg   (b) 2.5 tablets
   (c) Liquefy the tablets and add fluid to 250 cc.
6. (a) 25 cc   (b) 225 cc
7. (a) 200 cc   (b) 800 cc
8. (a) 25 cc   (b) 475 cc
9. (a) 3 tablets   (b) Liquefy the tablets and add fluid to 200 cc.
10. (a) $\frac{1}{4}$ (0.25) vial

    (b) Liquefy the powder and add fluid to 4 cc; you will have four doses of 0.125 mg/cc.
11. (a) $\frac{1}{5}$ (0.2) vial

    (b) Liquefy the powder and add fluid to 10 cc; you will have five doses of 200 mg per 2 cc.
12. (a) 125 cc   (b) 375 cc
13. (a) 9 cc   (b) 991 cc
14. (a) 50 cc   (b) 200 cc
15. (a) 3.5 g   (b) Fluid to 1000 cc
16. (a) 12.5 g   (b) Fluid to 500 cc
17. (a) 50 g   (b) Fluid to 250 cc

| **Drug Dosage Calculations Using the Apothecary System of Measurement**

12 | *Evaluation of Competency in the Use of Roman Numerals*

Self-assessment Test

The overall purpose of this section is self-evaluation of your competency with regard to roman numerals. The ability to use roman numerals is a necessary skill in order to use the apothecary system. Your general mathematics skills must also be good. You will, most certainly, need these skills to learn the apothecary system.

1. Write the following roman numerals in arabic numbers:
   a. LXIV
   b. xxvi
   c. CLXXV
   d. XI
   e. ii
   f. vii

2. Write the following arabic numbers in roman numerals:
   a. 39
   b. 1974
   c. 23
   d. 15
   e. 6
   f. 19

▶ Compare your answers with those located in the chapter's answer sheet. If you have answered all items correctly, you do not need a review. Bypass chapter 13. Otherwise, you are advised to proceed to the next chapter for review.

Answers for Chapter 12

1. a. 64
   b. 26
   c. 175
   d. 11
   e. 2
   f. 7
2. a. xxxix or XXXIX
   b. MCMLXXIV
   c. xxiii or XXIII
   d. xv or XV
   e. vi or VI
   f. xix or XIX

13 | *Review of Roman Numerals*

This system uses letters of the alphabet to designate or represent numbers. Although generally roman numerals are written using capital letters, health-related data are usually written using lower case letters. The following is a list of the basic roman numerals with the arabic equivalents:

Roman Numerals	Arabic Numbers
I or i	1
V or v	5
X or x	10
L or l	50
C or c	100
D or d	500
M or m	1000

Most numbers you will either have to write or interpret will be formed from a combination of the above letters.

There are a few basic rules that must be followed when writing roman numerals:

1. Roman numerals may be repeated. When they are it is like adding them. A roman numeral, however, *cannot* be repeated more than *three* times.

Example

iii is correct;   iiii is not correct.

Moreover, if a shorter written form is possible do not repeat letters, use the shorter form.

Example

vv = 10 is incorrect;   x = 10 is correct.
viv = 9 is incorrect;   ix = 9   is correct.

2. When a roman numeral is followed by one of lesser value, you add them to obtain the total value of the numbers

Example

$$\text{viii} = 5 + 1 + 1 + 1 = 8$$

3. When a roman numeral of lesser value is located before a higher value roman numeral, it is subtracted from that higher valued numeral.

Example

$$\text{iv} = 5 - 1 = 4$$

$$\text{xl} = 50 - 10 = 40$$

4. When a smaller valued numeral lies between two larger valued numerals, the small numeral is subtracted from the numeral that follows it

Example

$$\text{xix} = (10) + (10 - 1) = 10 + 9 = 19$$

$$\text{liv} = (50) + (5 - 1) = 50 + 4 = 54$$

▶   When you feel confident regarding this information, complete the practice problems that follow.

Practice Problems

Express the following arabic numbers as roman numerals:

1. 7	**2.** 29
3. 46	**4.** 15
5. 69	**6.** 13
7. 39	**8.** 25
9. 10	**10.** 24

Express the following roman numerals as arabic numbers:

11. xliv	**12.** xxxiii
13. xxvii	**14.** xiv
15. xi	**16.** xii
17. xxxviii	**18.** xlix
19. xvii	**20.** xliii

▶ Compare your answers with those in the answer sheet of this chapter. If you have answered all items correctly, you are ready to proceed to the next chapter. Otherwise, you should review the text and then correct your mistakes before proceeding to chapter 14.

Answers for Chapter 13

1. vii		2. xxix	
3. xlvi		4. xv	
5. lxix		6. xiii	
7. xxxix		8. xxv	
9. x		10. xxiv	
11. 44		12. 33	
13. 27		14. 14	
15. 11		16. 12	
17. 38		18. 49	
19. 17		20. 43	

14 | *Apothecary Measures*

TERMINAL PERFORMANCE OBJECTIVES

1. Given a fluid volume in the apothecary system, the reader is able to convert it into a larger or a number of smaller units equivalent in value.
2. Given a dosage of medication measured in grains in the apothecary system, the reader is able to calculate the number of solid preparations (pills) or the amount of liquid medication to be administered.
3. Given a selection of tablets or liquid preparations of various strength in the apothecary system, the reader is able to select the most appropriate strength and compute the number of tablets or the amount of liquid preparation to be administered.

INTERMEDIATE PERFORMANCE OBJECTIVES

After studying the text the reader is able to:

1. Define a minim.
2. Recognize from a given list and state the basic unit for fluid volume in the apothecary system.
3. Recognize from a given list and state the larger units for fluid volume in the apothecary system.
4. Write the abbreviation and symbol for the basic unit and larger units of fluid volume measures in the apothecary system.

5. Write the symbol for one-half in the apothecary system of measure.

6. State the meaning of a given symbol or abbreviation for the basic unit and larger units of fluid volume measures in the apothecary system.

7. State the meaning of $\overline{ss}$.

8. State the equivalent between the basic unit and larger units of fluid volume in the apothecary system.

9. Convert ounces to drams.

10. Convert drams to ounces or parts of an ounce.

11. Define grain.

12. Recognize and write the basic unit of weight in the apothecary system.

13. Recognize and write the abbreviation for the basic unit of weight in the apothecary system.

14. Recognize the existence of larger units of weight in the apothecary system.

15. Write dosage orders in the proper form.

16. Identify the active medication ingredient as opposed to the vehicle in which it is available.

17. Calculate the number of pills or volume of fluid to be administered.

► If you feel that you possess these skills, take the pretest. Otherwise begin to study the material in this chapter.

Pretest

1. (a) Define minim.   (b) Define grain.

2. The basic unit for fluid volume in the apothecary system is
   (a) grain   (b) minim   (c) gram
   (d) liter   (e) ounce   (f) dram
   (g) milliliter   (h) microgram   (i) cubic centimeter

3. Which of the following are units of fluid volume in the apothecary system?
   (a) grain   (b) dram   (c) ounce
   (d) cubic centimeter   (e) gram   (f) milliliter

4. Write the symbol and/or the abbreviation for the following:

	Symbol	*Abbreviation*
(a) one-half	_____	_____
(b) dram	_____	_____
(c) ounce	_____	_____
(d) fluid dram	_____	_____
(e) fluid ounce	_____	_____

5. The basic unit for weight in the apothecary system is
   (a) grain   (b) ounce   (c) dram
   (d) pound   (e) minim   (f) gram

6. Which of the following are units of weight in the apothecary system?
   (a) dram   (b) ounce   (c) gram
   (d) microgram   (e) milligram

7. Equivalents:
   (a) f℥ i ↔ ʒ _____   (b) ʒ i ↔ m _____   (c) 60 m ↔ ʒ _____

327

TPO   IPO

6

8. Write out the meaning for each abbreviation or symbol:
   (a) ʒ   (b) ʒ   (c) dr
   (d) m   (e) gr   (f) fʒ
   (g) $\overline{ss}$ (h) oz   (i) fʒ

9,10

9. Convert:
   (a) ʒ ii = ʒ _____   (b) ʒ XL = ʒ _____
   (c) 4 dr = _____ oz   (d) ʒ iii $\overline{ss}$ = _____ oz
   (e) ʒ xxxii = ʒ _____   (f) 2 dr = _____ oz

15

10. Although not always written as such, which of the following are written in the correct apothecary form?
    (a) ii ʒ   (b) gr x   (c) 4 gr   (d) ʒ iv $\overline{ss}$

16

11. Identify the active ingredient as opposed to the vehicle:
    (a) gr v in a ʒ   (b) An ʒ contains gr x
    (c) gr $\overline{ss}$ is in 5 m   (d) gr i $\overline{ss}$ is in ʒ $\overline{ss}$

2   9,10
      16,17

12. gr $\frac{1}{4}$ is 1 ʒ. You wish to give gr $\frac{1}{16}$.

    You will give ʒ _____ .

2   9,10
      16,17

13. You must give gr $\frac{1}{40}$. It is available as gr $\frac{1}{160}$ per ʒ.

    Give ʒ _____ .

2   9,10
      16,17

14. You must give ʒ i. The medication comes 240 gr/oz.
    You will give gr _____ .

2   9,10
      16,17

15. You must give gr 6. You have gr i $\overline{ss}$ per ʒ.
    You will give ʒ _____ .

2   9,10
      16,17

16. You must give gr $\frac{1}{120}$. You have gr $\frac{1}{30}$ per oz.

    You will give ʒ _____ .

3   16,17

17. You must administer gr $\frac{1}{150}$.

    You have available the following tablets:

    gr $\frac{1}{100}$, gr $\frac{1}{75}$, gr $\frac{1}{50}$, gr $\frac{1}{25}$, and gr $\frac{1}{15}$.

    You will give _____ .

TPO   IPO

3   9,10
     16,17

18. You must administer gr $\frac{1}{75}$.

    You have available the following oral liquid preparations:

    gr $\frac{1}{750}$ per ℥; gr $\frac{1}{15}$ per ℥; gr $\frac{1}{150}$ per ℥; gr $\frac{1}{25}$ per ℥; and

    gr $\frac{1}{75}$ per ℥ x.

    You will administer _____ .

▶ Compare your answers with those at the end of this chapter. If you have answered all questions correctly, continue to chapter 15. Otherwise, begin to study the material in this chapter before proceeding.

GENERAL INFORMATION

The apothecary system is a less exact system of measurement than the metric system. You will find in your practice that its usage is decreasing.

The active ingredient of medications in the apothecary system is generally measured in terms of a weight factor called a grain, and it is available in both dry and fluid vehicles. Common dry vehicles are pills, tablets, and capsules; apothecary fluid volume vehicles are measured in minims, drams, and ounces.

Every medication that you use will be labeled in terms of these two factors: the amount of active ingredient per vehicle. Two examples of labels for the apothecary system are given below.

1. 1 grain per dram
   Active ingredient: 1 grain
              Vehicle: 1 dram

2. 5 grains per tablet
   Active ingredient: 5 grains
              Vehicle: 1 tablet

Sometimes the labeling of a medication may combine both systems of measurement, such as 5 grains per 30 cc (5 grains is from the apothecary system, 30 cc from the metric system).

The apothecary system uses fractions rather than decimals for the writing of dosages, with the exception of the symbol $\overline{ss}$, which is used for one half. Roman numerals are used in this system when dosages are below 40. For dosages above 40 and for fractions arabic numbers are used.

In the apothecary system the basic units are the smaller ones, and the other units are larger and multiples of the basic unit. In writing the dosage order in the apothecary system the unit is written first, followed by the quantity, for example, gr 1/4.

Note that in discussions in this book drams refers to fluid drams and ounces refers to fluid ounces. Drams and ounces are mentioned in the section on weight so that you will recognize their existence. It is unlikely that you will ever be called upon to use them as a form of dry weight in calculating drug dosages, as they are too large a quantity.

When you are able to select a dosage from a varied assortment of preparations, the following should serve as your guide. For solid preparations choose the least amount and avoid any splitting of preparations; for liquid preparations choose a volume that is easily measurable. For oral liquids in the apothecary system the usual amount is between 1 and 8 drams. For intramuscular injections the usual amount is up to 32 minims and for subcutaneous injections up to 15 or 16 minims.

CONVERTING LIQUID MEASURES

	Abbreviations	Symbols	Equivalents
Basic unit			
Minim	m		
Larger units			
Dram	dr	ʒ = dram	
		fʒ = fluid dram	fʒ ↔ m 60
Ounce	oz	℥ = ounce	
		f℥ = fluid ounce	f℥ ↔ ʒ viii
		$\overline{ss} = \dfrac{1}{2}$	

Example

Calculate the number of drams in 2 oz:

$$2 \text{ oz} = \text{dr} _____$$

To Solve

We shall use the ratio–proportion method to solve this problem. (If necessary, review the section of chapter 4 in which this information was presented.) When using this method, the first relationship of the equation is obtained and established from the equivalents in the table above. Select the equivalent that contains a relationship of quantities that are the same quantities as those in the problem that you have to solve— here, ounces (℥) and drams (ʒ):

$$\frac{℥\,1}{ʒ\,8} = \frac{℥\,2}{ʒ\,x}$$

$$x = 2 \times 8$$

$$x = ʒ\,16$$

CONVERTING MEASURES OF WEIGHT

	Abbreviations	Symbols	Equivalents[a]
Basic unit			
Grain	gr, Gr		
Larger units			
Dram	dr	ʒ = dram	ʒ ↔ gr 60
Ounce	oz	ʒ = ounce	ʒ ↔ ʒ viii
		$\overline{ss} = \dfrac{1}{2}$	

[a] The equivalents of weights are rarely used, so do not memorize them.

Example

A drug comes as gr $\dfrac{1}{8}$ per dr 1 and you must give gr $\dfrac{1}{4}$.

To Solve

Dose on hand: gr $\dfrac{1}{8}$ per dr 1

Desired dose: gr $\dfrac{1}{4}$ per dr x

$$\frac{\text{gr } \dfrac{1}{8}}{\text{dr } 1} = \frac{\text{gr } \dfrac{1}{4}}{x}$$

$$\frac{1}{8} x = \frac{1}{4}$$

$$x = \frac{1}{4} \div \frac{1}{8}$$

$$x = \frac{1}{4} \times \frac{8}{1}$$

$$x = 2 \text{ dr}$$

▶   When you feel that you understand this material, complete the Activity Sheet.

Activity Sheet

1. The basic unit for weight in the apothecary system is
   - (a) gram
   - (b) ounce
   - (c) dram
   - (d) pound
   - (e) minim
   - (f) grain

2. The basic unit for fluid volume in the apothecary system is
   - (a) gram
   - (b) grain
   - (c) minim
   - (d) dram
   - (e) ounce
   - (f) liter
   - (g) milliliter

3. Which of the following are units of fluid volume in the apothecary system?
   - (a) grain
   - (b) dram
   - (c) ounce
   - (d) cubic centimeter
   - (e) gram

4. Which of the following are units of weight in the apothecary system?
   - (a) dram
   - (b) ounce
   - (c) gram
   - (d) milliliter
   - (e) liter

5. What is the basic unit of weight in the apothecary system?

6. What is the basic unit of fluid volume in the apothecary system?

7. Define minim.

8. Define grain.

9. Write out the meaning for each of the following abbreviations or symbols.
   - (a) ʒ = _____
   - (b) ℥ = _____
   - (c) dr = _____
   - (d) s̄s̄ = _____
   - (e) m = _____
   - (f) gr = _____
   - (g) fʒ = _____
   - (h) f℥ = _____
   - (i) oz = _____

10. Equivalents:
    - (a) fʒ 1 ↔ m _____
    - (b) f℥ 1 ↔ ʒ _____
    - (c) m 60 ↔ ʒ _____

333

11. Abbreviate:
    (a) grain = _____   (b) ounce = _____
    (c) dram = _____   (d) minim = _____

12. Write the symbol for:
    (a) ounce = _____   (b) dram = _____
    (c) one-half = _____   (d) fluid dram = _____
    (e) fluid ounce = _____

13. Mark T if the statement is true, F if the statement is false.
    (a) The words dram and ounce are often used interchangeably
        for fluid dram and fluid ounce, respectively.
    (b) Rarely will you use the units drams and ounce for the weight
        of medications because these units are too large.
    (c) In the apothecary system quantities under 40 are usually
        expressed in roman numerals.
    (d) In the apothecary system quantities over 40 and most frac-
        tions are expressed in arabic numbers.
    (e) In expressing dosages in the apothecary system the quantity
        is written after the unit, such as gr v rather than v gr.

14. The abbreviation(s) for grain is/are
    (a) G   (b) Gm   (c) Gr
    (d) gr   (e) g

15. The minim is a small unit of fluid volume in the apothecary
    system. What are the larger units?

16. f℥ 8 = f℥ _____

17. f℥ 6 = ℥ _____

18. f℥ 16 = f℥ _____

19. f℥ $\frac{1}{2}$ = f℥ _____

20. ℥ $\frac{3}{4}$ = ℥ _____

21. ℥ 4 = dr _____

22. $\frac{1}{4}$ oz = dr _____

23. 3 oz = dr _____

24. $\dfrac{1}{8}$ oz = dr _____

25. ℥ vii = oz _____

26. 2$\dfrac{3}{4}$ oz = ℥ _____

27. Write $\dfrac{1}{2}$ grain in apothecary form.

28. Write 3 grains in apothecary form.

29. Write 1$\dfrac{1}{2}$ grains in apothecary form.

30. Write 30 grains in apothecary form.

31. Write $\dfrac{1}{120}$ grain in apothecary form.

32. Select the medication component and the vehicle in the following items:
    (a) gr v per capsule   (b) gr x per ℥   (c) gr i per m
    (d) gr vi per tablet   (e) gr x per cc

33. Tablets available are gr 1/4 and you must administer gr $\overline{ss}$. You give _____ tablet(s).

34. You have tablets gr 1/150 available and you must administer gr 1/300. You will give _____ tablet(s).

35. You must administer gr iii and the capsules available are gr i $\overline{ss}$. You will give _____ capsule(s).

36. You must prepare gr xx of a medication and the available capsules are gr v. You will administer _____ capsule(s).

37. You must administer gr vii $\overline{ss}$ and your tablets are available as gr xv. You will give _____ tablet(s).

38. A medication comes as gr 1/4 per ℥ and you must administer gr 1/8. You will administer dram(s) _____ .

39. You must prepare gr 1/32 and the medication comes gr 1/16 pe 3. You will give ounce(s) _____ .

40. You must administer gr 1/100 and the dosage available is g 1/200 per 3. You will give dram(s) _____ .

41. The order reads: "Administer gr i s̄s̄," and your tablets are gr 3/4 each. You will give _____ tablet(s).

42. The order reads: "Administer gr 1/40," and your tablets are gr 1/120. You will give _____ tablet(s).

43. A medicine comes gr 1/20 per ounce and you must administer gr 1/80. How much will you give the person (a) in ounces (b) ir drams?

44. A medicine is available as gr s̄s̄ per oz and you must give gr 1/8. How many drams will you give?

45. When you are able to select from different strength preparations. what should serve as your guide in the selection of a dose for solid preparations?

46. List the usual amount of liquid medication administered in the apothecary system for the following routes:
(a) oral   (b) injection

47. You must administer gr 1/150. You have available the following grain tablets: 1/50, 1/75, 1/100, 1/200, and 1/300. You will give _____ .

48. You must administer gr 1/8. You have available the following oral liquid preparations; gr 1/2 per dr, gr 1/4 per dr, gr 1/16 per dr, and gr 1/16 per oz. You will administer _____ .

49. You must administer gr 1/16. You have available the following grain capsules: 1/2, 1/4, 1/8, 1/1.6, and 1/32. You will administer _____ .

50. You must administer gr 1/60. You have available the following liquid oral preparations: gr 1/10 per 3, gr 1/20 per 3, gr 1/30 per 3, gr 1/120 per 3. You will administer _____ .

▶ Compare your answers with those at the end of this chapter. If you have answered all questions correctly, take the posttest. Otherwise, review the preceding text and correct your mistakes before taking the posttest.

Posttest

<table>
<tr><td>TPO</td><td>IPO</td><td></td></tr>
<tr><td></td><td>1,11</td><td>1. Define (a) minim and (b) grain.</td></tr>
</table>

TPO — IPO

1,11

1. Define (a) minim and (b) grain.

2

2. The basic unit for fluid volume in the apothecary system is
   (a) grain   (b) minim   (c) gram
   (d) liter   (e) ounce   (f) dram
   (g) milliliter   (h) microgram   (i) cubic centimeter

3

3. Which of the following are units of fluid volume in the apothecary system?
   (a) grain   (b) dram   (c) ounce
   (d) cubic centimeter   (e) gram   (f) milliliter

4,5

4. Write the symbol and/or the abbreviation for the following:

	Symbol	*Abbreviation*
(a) one half	_____	_____
(b) dram	_____	_____
(c) ounce	_____	_____
(d) fluid dram	_____	_____
(e) fluid ounce	_____	_____

12

5. The basic unit for weight in the apothecary system is
   (a) grain   (b) ounce   (c) dram
   (d) pound   (e) minim   (f) gram

13,14

6. Which of the following are units of weight in the apothecary system:
   (a) dram   (b) ounce   (c) gram
   (d) microgram   (e) milligram

8

7. Equivalents:
   (a) f℥ i ↔ m _____   (b) f℥ ↔ ℥ _____   (c) m 60 ↔ ℥ _____

6

8. Write out the meaning for the following:
   (a) dr   (b) m   (c) $\mathfrak{z}$
   (d) $\mathfrak{z}$ (e) gr   (f) f$\mathfrak{z}$
   (g) f$\mathfrak{z}$ (h) oz   (i) $\overline{\text{ss}}$

9,10

9. Convert:
   (a) $\mathfrak{z}$ i $\overline{\text{ss}}$ = $\mathfrak{z}$ _____   (b) $\mathfrak{z}$ xxiv = $\mathfrak{z}$ _____
   (c) 1 dr = _____ oz   (d) v oz = _____ dr
   (e) $\mathfrak{z}$ xvi = $\mathfrak{z}$ _____   (f) 6 dr = _____ oz

15

10. Although not always written as such, which of the following are in correct apothecary form?
    (a) $\mathfrak{z}$ i $\overline{\text{ss}}$ (b) V $\mathfrak{z}$ (c) Gr X   (d) VI Gr

16

11. Identify the active ingredient as opposed to the vehicle:
    (a) gr XX per $\mathfrak{z}$ V   (b) $\mathfrak{z}$ $\overline{\text{ss}}$ contains gr X
    (c) gr i $\overline{\text{ss}}$ is in 30 m   (d) gr 1/4 is in a $\mathfrak{z}$

2   9,10
           16,17

12. gr 1/3 is in 1 $\mathfrak{z}$. You wish to give gr 1/12. You will give $\mathfrak{z}$ _____ .

2   9,10
           16,17

13. You must give gr 1/30. It comes as gr 1/120 per $\mathfrak{z}$. You will give _____ oz.

2   9,10
           16,17

14. You must give $\mathfrak{z}$ i. The medicine comes 480 gr/oz. You will give gr _____ .

2   9,10
           16,17

15. You must give gr iii. You have gr 3/4 per $\mathfrak{z}$. You will give $\mathfrak{z}$ _____ .

2   9,10
           16,17

16. You must give gr 1/80. You have gr 1/20 per oz. You will give $\mathfrak{z}$ _____ .

3   16,17

17. You must administer gr 1/240. You have available the following grain tablets: 1/24, 1/48, 1/120, 1/480, and 1/80. You will administer _____ .

18. You must administer gr 1/40. You have available the following oral liquid preparations:

$$\text{gr } \frac{1}{160} \text{ per } \mathfrak{z}, \text{ gr } \frac{1}{160} \text{ per } \mathfrak{z}, \text{ gr } \frac{1}{40} \text{ per } \mathfrak{z} \text{ x,}$$

$$\text{gr } \frac{1}{20} \text{ per } \mathfrak{z}, \text{ and gr } \frac{1}{10} \text{ per } \mathfrak{z};$$

You would administer _____ .

▶ Compare your answers with those at the end of this chapter. If you have answered all questions correctly, continue to chapter 15. Otherwise, note the objective numbers beside the problems that you have answered incorrectly, review the relevant text, and practice the appropriate items on the activity sheet. Then correct your mistakes on the posttest and take the pretest as a second posttest before continuing to chapter 15.

Answers for Chapter 14

PRETEST

1. (a) Smallest, basic unit of liquid measure in the apothecary system
   (b) Smallest, basic unit of weight in the apothecary system
2. (b)
3. (b), (c)
4. (a) $\overline{ss}$ (b) ʒ, dr   (c) ℥, oz   (d) fʒ   (e) f℥
5. (a)
6. (a) and (b)
7. (a) viii   (b) 60   (c) i
8. (a) dram   (b) ounce   (c) dram   (d) minim   (e) grain
   (f) fluid dram   (g) $\frac{1}{2}$ (h) ounce   (i) fluid ounce
9. (a) 16   (b) 5   (c) $\overline{ss}$ (d) 28   (e) 4   (f) $\frac{1}{4}$
10. (b) and (d)
11. | **Active Ingredient** | **Vehicle** |
    | --- | --- |
    | (a) gr v | ʒ |
    | (b) gr x | ℥ |
    | (c) gr $\overline{ss}$ | m 5 |
    | (d) gr i $\overline{ss}$ | ʒ $\overline{ss}$ |
12. 2
13. $\frac{1}{2}$ or $\overline{ss}$
14. 30
15. $\frac{1}{2}$ or $\overline{ss}$
16. 2
17. One half of the gr $\frac{1}{75}$ tablet
18. ʒ ii of gr $\frac{1}{150}$ per ʒ

340

CTIVITY SHEET

1. (f)
2. (c)
3. (b) and (c)
4. (a) and (b)
5. Grain
6. Minim
7. Smallest and basic unit of fluid volume in the apothecary system
8. Smallest and basic unit of weight in the apothecary system
9. (a) dram   (b) ounce   (c) dram   (d) one-half   (e) minim
     (f) grain   (g) fluid dram   (h) fluid ounce   (i) ounce
10. (a) 60   (b) 8   (c) 1
11. (a) gr, Gr   (b) oz   (c) dr   (d) m
12. (a) ʒ   (b) ℥   (c) s̅s̅   (d) fʒ   (e) f℥
13. (a) T   (b) T   (c) T   (d) T   (e) T
14. (d) and (c)
15. Dram and ounce

16. 1	17. $\frac{3}{4}$	18. 128
19. 4	20. 6	21. 32
22. 2	23. 24	24. 1
25. $\frac{7}{8}$	26. 22	27. gr s̅s̅
28. gr iii	29. gr i s̅s̅	30. gr xxx
31. gr $\frac{1}{120}$		

32.

Medication	**Vehicle**
(a) gr v	capsule
(b) gr x	ʒ
(c) gr i	m
(d) gr vi	tablet
(e) gr x	cc

33. 2	34. $\frac{1}{2}$ or s̅s̅	35. 2
36. 4	37. $\frac{1}{2}$ or s̅s̅	38. $\frac{1}{2}$ or s̅s̅
39. $\frac{1}{2}$ or s̅s̅	40. 2	41. 2

42. 3   43. (a) $\frac{1}{4}$ (b) 2   44. 2

45. (a) Use the least amount.   (b) Avoid split tablets.

46. (a) 1 to 8 drams   (b) Up to 32 minims

47. Two gr $\frac{1}{300}$ tablets   48. 2 dr of gr $\frac{1}{16}$

49. Two gr $\frac{1}{32}$ tablets   50. ℨ ii of gr $\frac{1}{120}$

POSTTEST

1. (a) Smallest and basic unit of liquid measure in the apothecary system
   (b) Smallest and basic unit of weight in the apothecary system
2. (b)
3. (b) and (c)
4. (a) $\overline{ss}$ (b) ℨ, dr   (c) ℨ, oz   (d) f ℨ   (e) f ℥
5. (a)
6. (a) and (b)
7. (a) 60   (b) viii   (c) i
8. (a) Dram   (b) Minim   (c) Ounce   (d) Dram   (e) Grain
   (f) Fluid dram   (g) Fluid ounce   (h) Ounce   (i) $\frac{1}{2}$
9. (a) 12   (b) 3   (c) $\frac{1}{8}$ (d) 40   (e) 2   (f) $\frac{3}{4}$
10. (a) and (c)
11. **Active Ingredient**   **Vehicle**
    (a) gr xx   ℨ V
    (b) gr X   ℥ $\overline{ss}$
    (c) gr i $\overline{ss}$ 30 m
    (d) gr $\frac{1}{4}$ ℨ

12. 2   13. $\frac{1}{2}$ or $\overline{ss}$ 14. 60   15. $\frac{1}{2}$ or $\overline{ss}$

16. 2   17. 2 of the $\frac{1}{480}$ 18. ℨ iv or ℥ $\overline{ss}$ of gr $\frac{1}{160}$ per ℨ

15 | *Conversion Among Metric, Apothecary, and Household Measures*

TERMINAL PERFORMANCE OBJECTIVES

1. Given a dosage in the apothecary system, the reader is able to convert it into the metric system, and vice versa, and calculate the number of tablets or the amount of fluid volume to administer.
2. Given a choice of various preparations in the apothecary and the metric systems, the reader is able to select the most appropriate preparation and calculate the amount to be administered.

INTERMEDIATE PERFORMANCE OBJECTIVES

After studying the text, the reader is able to:

1. State the conversion factors between the apothecary and the metric systems of fluid volume.
2. State the fluid volume equivalent for a given quantity in the opposite system.
3. Convert cubic centimeters to minims.
4. Convert minims to cubic centimeters.
5. Convert cubic centimeters to drams.
6. Convert drams to cubic centimeters.
7. Convert cubic centimeters to ounces.

▶ Do not attempt this chapter until you have completed the chapters on metric measures, conversion between metric and household measures, and apothecary measures.

8. Convert ounces to cubic centimeters.

9. Compute the amount of fluid volume to administer for a ca[l]culated dosage.

10. Compute the amount of medication you are giving when yo[u] have facts concerning the fluid volume to be administered an[d] the amount of medication per unit volume.

11. State the equivalent for a given liquid measure in the apothe[-]cary, metric, or household system.

12. State the equivalent conversion factors among household, apoth[-]ecary, and metric measures of fluid volume.

13. Convert teaspoons to cubic centimeters.

14. Convert teaspoons to drams.

15. Convert cubic centimeters to teaspoons.

16. Convert drams to teaspoons.

17. Convert tablespoons to drams.

18. Convert tablespoons to cubic centimeters.

19. Convert drams to tablespoons.

20. Convert cubic centimeters to tablespoons.

21. Convert ounces to cubic centimeters.

22. Convert cubic centimeters to ounces.

23. Compute the amount of fluid volume to be administered in either apothecary, metric, or household measures for a prescribed dosage.

24. Compute the amount of medication that is to be administered from a specified fluid volume.

25. State the equivalent conversion factors for converting weight between the apothecary and metric systems.

26. State the two guides for converting weight between the apothecary and metric systems.

27. List the six equivalent conversion factors that are exceptions to the two guides for converting measures of weight between the apothecary and metric systems.

28. Convert grains to milligrams.

29. Convert milligrams to grains.

30. Convert grains to grams.

31. Convert grams to grains.

32. Convert a given dosage in one system to its equivalent in the other system and then calculate the number of tablets or the fluid volume in any system to be administered.

▶   If you feel that you possess these skills, take the pretest. Otherwise, begin to study the material in this chapter.

Pretest

TPO   IPO

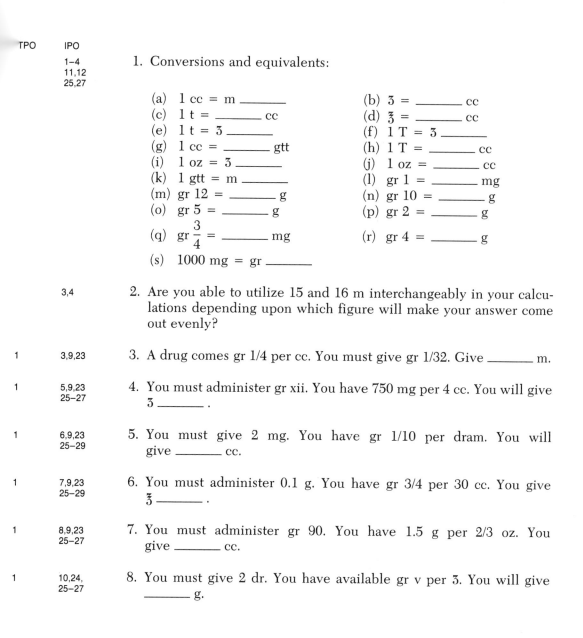

1–4
11,12
25,27

1. Conversions and equivalents:

    (a) 1 cc = m _____   (b) ℥ = _____ cc

    (c) 1 t = _____ cc   (d) ℨ = _____ cc

    (e) 1 t = ℨ _____   (f) 1 T = ℨ _____

    (g) 1 cc = _____ gtt   (h) 1 T = _____ cc

    (i) 1 oz = ℨ _____   (j) 1 oz = _____ cc

    (k) 1 gtt = m _____   (l) gr 1 = _____ mg

    (m) gr 12 = _____ g   (n) gr 10 = _____ g

    (o) gr 5 = _____ g   (p) gr 2 = _____ g

    (q) gr $\dfrac{3}{4}$ = _____ mg   (r) gr 4 = _____ g

    (s) 1000 mg = gr _____

3,4

2. Are you able to utilize 15 and 16 m interchangeably in your calculations depending upon which figure will make your answer come out evenly?

1   3,9,23

3. A drug comes gr 1/4 per cc. You must give gr 1/32. Give _____ m.

1   5,9,23
25–27

4. You must administer gr xii. You have 750 mg per 4 cc. You will give ℨ _____ .

1   6,9,23
25–29

5. You must give 2 mg. You have gr 1/10 per dram. You will give _____ cc.

1   7,9,23
25–29

6. You must administer 0.1 g. You have gr 3/4 per 30 cc. You give ℨ _____ .

1   8,9,23
25–27

7. You must administer gr 90. You have 1.5 g per 2/3 oz. You give _____ cc.

1   10,24,
25–27

8. You must give 2 dr. You have available gr v per ℨ. You will give _____ g.

TPO	IPO	
1	7,8,10 24–27, 30,31	9. You must give 30 cc. The medication is available as gr vii $\overline{ss}$ per ℥ $\overline{ss}$. You will give _____ mg.
1	13,23, 25–27	10. You must administer gr iv. You have available 250 mg/t. You will give _____ cc.
1	14,23, 25–29	11. You have available 0.1 mg/t. You must administer gr 1/150. You will give ℥ _____ .
1	15,23, 25–29	12. You have available gr 1/12 per 2 cc. You must administer 25 mg. You will give _____ t.
1	16,23, 25–29	13. You must administer 1 mg. You have available gr 1/300 per ℥. You will give _____ t.
1	17,23, 25–29	14. You have available gr 1/30 per T. You must administer 1 mg. You will give ℥ _____ .
1	18,23, 25–27, 30,31	15. You have available 500 mg/T. You must administer gr xxii $\overline{ss}$. You will give _____ cc.
1	19,23, 25–31	16. You have available gr 1/300 per dr. You must administer 1.2 mg. You will give _____ T.
1	20,23, 25–27, 30,31	17. You have available gr i $\overline{ss}$ per 45 cc. You must administer 0.1 g. You will give _____ T.
1	21,23, 25–27	18. You must administer 250 mg. You have available gr ii per oz. You will give _____ cc.
1	22,23, 25–27	19. There are gr x per 30 cc. You must administer 0.3 g. You will give ℥ _____ .
1	25–29,32	20. You have available gr 1/120 tablets. You must administer 0.25 mg. You will give _____ tablets.

TPO	IPO	
1	25–27, 30–32	21. You have available 0.5 g per tablet. You must administer gr xxxvii s͞s. You will give _____ tablets.
1	25–27,32	22. You must administer 0.05 g. You have available gr 3/4 per tablet. You will give _____ tablets.
2	25–29,32	23. You must administer 15 mg. You have available the following tablets: 3 mg, gr 1/4, gr s͞s, 30 mg, and gr i. The most appropriate dose would be _____ tablet(s) of the _____ strength.
2	25–29, 32	24. You must administer gr 1/150. You have available the following tablets: gr 1/75, gr 1/300, 0.2 mg, 0.4 mg, and 0.8 mg. The most appropriate dose would be _____ tablet(s) of the _____ strength.

▶ Compare your answers with those at the end of the chapter. If you have answered all questions correctly, you may bypass this chapter. Otherwise, begin to study the text that follows.

CONVERTING LIQUID MEASURES FROM THE APOTHECARY TO THE METRIC SYSTEM

> **Equivalent Conversion Factors**
> m 15–16 ↔ 1 cc
>
> ℥ i ↔ 4 cc
>
> ℥ i ↔ 30 cc

There are no exact equivalents; these are just approximations. You should readily see the discrepancy. It is said 1 dr = 4 cc and oz 1 = 30 cc. If, however, you multiply 8 dr by 4 cc per dram, you obtain 32 cc. A good compromise is to use 30 cc when converting ounces and 4 cc when converting drams except when you see dr 8. Think of dr 8 as 1 oz and therefore 30 cc. Think of dr 4 as 1/2 oz or 15 cc.

Example

℥ xxxiv = _____ cc.

To Solve
The first relationship in the equation comes from conversion factors.

$$\frac{℥\ i}{30\ cc} = \frac{℥\ 34}{x\ cc}$$

$$x = 30 \times 34$$

$$x = 1020\ cc$$

Example

If a medication comes as gr 1/3 per ℥ and you must give gr 1/6, how many cc will you give?

$$\text{Dose on hand: gr } \frac{1}{3} \text{ per ℥ (or 30 cc)}$$

$$\text{Desired dose: gr } \frac{1}{6}$$

To Solve
You can solve two ways: (A) start with the given fluid volume ℥ i and then convert to cubic centimeters at the end of the problem, or (B) substitute the known cc volume for the given fluid volume—℥ i ↔ 30 cc—and solve for cc.

Method A

$$\frac{\text{gr} \frac{1}{3}}{\text{Ʒ} \, 1} = \frac{\text{gr} \frac{1}{6}}{\text{Ʒ} \, x}$$

$$\frac{1}{3} x = \frac{1}{6}$$

$$x = \frac{1}{6} \div \frac{1}{3}$$

$$x = \frac{1}{6} \times 3$$

$$x = \frac{1}{2} \, \text{Ʒ}$$

$$x = 15 \text{ cc}$$

Method B

$$\frac{\text{gr} \frac{1}{3}}{30 \text{ cc}} = \frac{\text{gr} \frac{1}{6}}{x \text{ cc}}$$

$$\frac{1}{3} x = \frac{1}{6} \times 30$$

$$\frac{1}{3} x = 5$$

$$x = 5 \div \frac{1}{3}$$

$$x = 5 \times 3$$

$$x = 15 \text{ cc}$$

▶   When you feel that you understand this material, complete Activity Sheet 1.

Activity Sheet 1

For questions 1 through 18, convert or state the equivalent for the units indicated.

1. ℥ i = _____ cc

2. ʒ i _____ cc

3. 1 cc = m _____

4. 2 cc = m _____

5. 10 cc = ʒ _____

6. 0.25 mL = m _____

7. $\frac{2}{3}$ cc = m _____

8. 300 cc = ℥ _____

9. 2 cc = ʒ _____

10. 20 cc = ʒ _____

11. ℥ iv ʒ ii = _____ mL

12. ℥ iii s̄s̄ = _____ cc

13. 76 cc = ʒ _____

14. 25 m = _____ cc

15. 15 cc = ʒ _____

16. ℥ ii s̄s̄ = _____ cc

17. ʒ ii s̄s̄ = _____ mL

18. 45 cc = ℥ _____

19. A drug is available as gr 1/6 per ℥ and you must administer gr 1/18. How many cubic centimeters is this?

20. A drug is available as gr ii per ʒ and you must administer ʒ ii s̄s̄. How many grains is this?

21. A drug is available as gr v per ʒ and you must administer 20 cc. How many grains of medication will you give?

22. A medication is available as gr x per 15 cc and you must administer gr xxx. How much will you give in ounces?

23. A drug is available as gr 1/260 per 5 cc and you must administer gr 1/65. How much will you administer in ʒ?

24. A drug is available as 0.6 g/℥. You must administer 20 mg. How much will you administer in cubic centimeters?

25. A drug is available as 36 mg/cc and you must administer 1.62 g. How much fluid volume will you give in ℥?

26. A medicine is available as 50 mcg/cc and you must administer 0.4 mg. How much will you administer in ℥?

27. You must administer ʒ vi and the medication available is 35 mcg/cc. How many milligrams will you administer?

► Compare your answers with those at the end of the chapter. If you have answered all questions correctly, continue to the next section of text. Otherwise, review the preceding text and correct your mistakes before proceeding.

CONVERTING LIQUID MEASURES FROM THE METRIC TO THE APOTHECARY SYSTEM

Fractional parts of a cubic centimeter (or milliliter) are utilized when you are giving injections. Some syringes have two scales on them, as shown in the figure below. One side is metric and measured in tenths of a cubic centimeter. The other scale is apothecary and measured in minims. When a dose you desire to give does not measure out evenly in tenths of a cubic centimeter, you may have to measure it in minims. For example, 0.1, 0.2, 0.3, and 1.3 cc can be measured, whereas $\frac{2}{3}$ and $\frac{1}{3}$ cc cannot be measured.

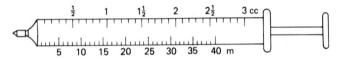

A typical small syringe (2 to 3 cc). Larger ones are calibrated differently and lack measurement in minims.

To convert between minims and cubic centimeters (or milliliters), use the conversion factor: 1 cc = 15 or 16 m. The 15 and 16 m are interchangeable; use the conversion factor that will make your calculations come out to an even number, that is, when converting $\frac{1}{3}$ cc use 15 m, and with $\frac{1}{4}$ cc use 16 m.

Example

You must give 50 mg of a drug and it is available as 40 mg/cc. How much will you give?

Dose on hand: 40 mg/cc

Desired dose: 50 mg

To Solve
Determine what part of a cubic centimeter you must give. Then use the conversion factor that makes minims come out evenly. (Here 16 m is used because it divides evenly: $\frac{1}{4}$ cc = 4 m.)

$$\frac{40 \text{ mg}}{1 \text{ cc}} = \frac{50}{x}$$

$$40x = 50$$

$$x = \frac{5\emptyset}{4\emptyset}$$

$$x = 1\frac{1}{4} \text{ cc}$$

We now convert $1\frac{1}{4}$ cc to minims

$$\frac{16 \text{ m}}{1 \text{ cc}} = \frac{x \text{ m}}{1\frac{1}{4} \text{ cc}}$$

$$x = 16 \times 1\frac{1}{4}$$

$$x = 16 \times \frac{5}{4}$$

$$x = \overset{4}{\cancel{16}} \times \frac{5}{\underset{1}{\cancel{4}}}$$

$$x = 20 \text{ m}$$

▶   When you feel that you understand this material, complete Activity Sheet 2.

Activity Sheet 2

1. A medication comes gr 1/8 per cc and you must administer gr 1/24. You will give m _____ .

2. A medication comes 50 mg/cc and you must administer 62.5 mg. You will give m _____ .

3. A medication is available as gr 1/75 per cc. You must prepare gr 1/100. You will give m _____ .

4. A drug preparation is 0.75 g/cc and you must administer 500 mg. You will give m _____ .

5. You must administer 35 mcg. The medicine is available as 0.14 mg/cc. You will give m _____ .

6. A medication preparation is labeled 750 mg/cc and you must administer 1 g. You will give m _____ .

7. A drug is available as gr 1/2 per cc and you must administer gr 7/8. You will give m _____ .

8. You must administer 0.15 g and the medication available is 600 mg/cc. You will give m _____ .

9. You must administer gr 5/9. It is available as gr 1/3 per cc. You will give m _____ .

10. A drug is available 0.5 mg/cc and you must administer 0.125 mg. You will give m _____ .

▶ Compare your answers with those at the end of the chapter. If you have answered all questions correctly, continue to the next section of text. Otherwise, review the preceding text and correct your mistakes before proceeding.

CONVERTING LIQUID MEASURES AMONG THE METRIC, APOTHECARY, AND HOUSEHOLD MEASURES

Household Measures	Apothecary	Metric
15–16 gtt	= m 15–16	= 1 cc
1 t	$= 3 \text{ i} \frac{1}{4}$	= 5 cc
1 T	= 3 iv	= 15 cc
1 oz	= dr 8 (1 oz)	= 30 cc

These are the measures you will find being used in most of the clinical areas where you will be practicing. The figure below illustrates a typical medicine cup calibrated with these measures.

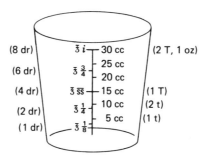

A sample medicine cup

Example

$$2 \text{ t} = 3 \underline{\hspace{2cm}} = \underline{\hspace{2cm}} \text{cc.}$$

To Solve
Use the equivalents to set up the first relationship in the equation:

Household to Apothecary

$$\frac{1 \text{ t}}{3 \, 1\frac{1}{4}} = \frac{2 \text{ t}}{3 \, x}$$

$$x = 2 \times 1\frac{1}{4}$$

$$x = 2 \times \frac{5}{4}$$

$$x = 3 \, 2\frac{1}{2}$$

Household to Metric

$$\frac{1 \text{ t}}{5 \text{ cc}} = \frac{2 \text{ t}}{x \text{ cc}}$$

$$x = 5 \times 2$$

$$x = 10 \text{ cc}$$

Example

A medication comes gr 1/27 per 5 cc and you must give gr 1/9. How much will you give in household measure?

To Solve

We first determine the amount in cc and then convert to household measure.

$$\frac{\text{gr} \frac{1}{27}}{5 \text{ cc}} = \frac{\text{gr} \frac{1}{9}}{x \text{ cc}}$$

$$\frac{1}{27} x = 5 \times \frac{1}{9}$$

$$x = 5 \times \frac{1}{9} \div \frac{1}{27}$$

$$x = 5 \times \frac{1}{9} \times \frac{27}{1}$$

$$x = 15 \text{ cc}$$

We do not need to set up a second equation to convert cc to household measure because we already know, from the table of equivalents, that 15 cc = 1 T.

▶   When you feel that you understand this material, complete Activity Sheet 3.

Activity Sheet 3

For questions 1 through 19, convert or state the equivalent for the units indicated.

1. gtt = m _____

2. 1 cc = _____ gtt

3. 1 T = 3 _____ = _____ cc

4. 30 cc = _____ oz

5. 15 cc = 3 _____

6. 8 dr = _____ oz = _____ cc

7. 5 cc = 3 _____ = _____ t

8. 8 t = 3 _____

9. 45 cc = _____ t

10. 5 dr = _____ t

11. 2 T = dr _____

12. 3 T = _____ cc

13. 4 dr = _____ T

14. 75 cc _____ T

15. $2\frac{1}{2}$ oz = _____ cc

16. $3\frac{1}{5}$ t = _____ cc

17. 120 t = dr _____

18. 8 oz = _____ cc

19. 150 cc = _____ oz

20. You must give gr 5/8 and you have available gr 1/4 per 3. How much will you give in household measure?

21. You have available gr 1/120 per 5 cc and you must administer gr 1/40. You will give _____ t.

22. A medication comes 0.5 g per 60 cc and you must give 125 mg. You will give _____ T.

23. You have available 0.66 g per 30 cc and you must administer 1 t. How many milligrams will you give?

24. You must administer 1 t of a drug and your available stock is 500 mg per 30 cc. How many milligrams will you give?

25. A medicine is ordered as gr 1/150. You have gr 1/300 per 0.5 cc. How will you give this dose in household measure?

26. A medicine is available as 225 mg per oz $\overline{ss}$ and you must give 75 mg. You will give how much in household measure?

27. A drug comes as 22 mg per 3 and you must give 132 mg. You will give how much in household measure?

28. A drug comes as 45 mcg/cc and you must administer 0.45 mg. How much will you give in household measure?

29. A drug is available as 1.2 g/oz and you must give 300 mg. You will give _____ T.

▶ Compare your answers with those at the end of the chapter. If you have answered all questions correctly, continue to the next section of text. Otherwise, review the previous text and correct your mistakes before proceeding.

CONVERTING MEASURES OF WEIGHT BETWEEN APOTHECARY AND METRIC MEASURES

Equivalent Conversion Factors	Exceptions to Guides
gr 1 ↔ 60 mg	gr 12 = 750 mg (0.75 g)
gr 15 ↔ 1 g (1000 mg)	gr 10 = 600 mg (0.6 g)
	gr 5 = 300 mg (0.3 g)
	gr 4 = 250 mg (0.25 g)
	gr 2 = 120 mg (0.12 g)
	gr $\frac{3}{4}$ = 45 or 50 mg

The following guides will prevent you from needing to memorize long lists of equivalents, such as you will see in many books:

1. If the quantity you are converting is gr 1 (60 mg) or less, use the equivalent 60 mg = gr 1.
2. If the quantity you are converting is more than gr 1 (60 mg), use the equivalent gr 15 = 1 g (1000 mg).

The six exceptions to these guides are listed in the table above. These should be memorized.

Example

$$\text{gr } \frac{1}{300} = \text{_____ mg.}$$

To Solve

This is not an exception. Since the amount is less than gr 1, we use the equivalent gr 1 = 60 mg. The equivalent conversion factor is the first relationship in the equation.

$$\frac{60 \text{ mg}}{\text{gr } 1} = \frac{x}{\text{gr } \frac{1}{300}}$$

$$x = 60 \times \frac{1}{300} = \frac{\overset{1}{\cancel{60}}}{1} \times \frac{1}{\underset{5}{\cancel{300}}}$$

$$x = \frac{1}{5} \text{ or } 0.2 \text{ mg}$$

Example

gr 45 = _____ mg.

To Solve

This is not an exception. Since the amount is more than 1 gr use the equivalent 15 gr = 1 g (1000 mg). The equivalent conversion factor is the first relationship in the equation.

$$\frac{\text{gr } 15}{1000 \text{ mg}} = \frac{\text{gr } 45}{x}$$

$$15x = 45 \times 1000$$

$$15x = 45,000$$

$$x = 45,000 \div 15$$

$$x = 3000 \text{ mg}$$

► When you feel that you understand this material, complete Activity Sheet 4.

Activity Sheet 4

1. State the two guides to be utilized in converting weight between the apothecary and metric systems.

2. List the six equivalent conversion factors that are exceptions to the two guides you stated in the previous question.

3. 750 mg = _____ g = gr _____

4. gr $\dfrac{1}{4}$ = _____ mg

5. gr $\dfrac{1}{200}$ = _____ mg

6. gr $\dfrac{1}{150}$ = _____ mg

7. gr $\dfrac{1}{60}$ = _____ mg

8. gr iv = _____ mg

9. 100 mg = _____ g = gr _____

10. 2 g = gr _____

11. 120 mg = gr _____

12. gr v = _____ g = _____ mg

13. gr vii $\overline{ss}$ = _____ g = _____ mg

14. gr XV = _____ g = _____ mg

15. 40 mg = gr _____

16. 7.5 mg = gr _____

17. 0.5 mg = gr _____

18. 50 mg = gr _____

19. gr $\dfrac{3}{4}$ = _____ mg

20. 10 mg = gr _____

▶ Compare your answers with those at the end of the chapter. If you have answered all questions correctly, continue to the next section of text. Otherwise, review the previous text and then correct your mistakes before proceeding.

GUIDE TO SOLVING CONVERSION PROBLEMS

Example

A medication is available as 0.2 mg per 4 cc and you must administer gr 1/75. How much will you administer in drams?

To Solve

1. Identify what quantities are available and what are desired.

Dose available: 0.2 mg per 4 cc

Desired dose: $\text{gr } \dfrac{1}{75}$ per dr _____

Be sure to organize these data so that the active ingredient is to one side and the vehicle is to the other. The missing quantity becomes x, and its value is the solution to the problem.

2. Inspect the quantities. Ask yourself the following:
   (a) Are the active ingredients in the same system: Remember these must not only be in the same system but the quantities must be within the same specific level of value within the same system in order to solve the problem.
   (b) Are the vehicles the same? (This question is especially significant with regard to liquid measures, where both the system and the level of value within the system can vary.)
   In the present example both systems are present.

Active Ingredient	Vehicle
0.2 mg—metric system	4 cc—metric system
$\text{gr } \dfrac{1}{75}$—apothecary system	dr—apothecary system

3. Convert as necessary.

   The quantities of the active ingredient must be either both in milligrams or both in grains. Either conversion is acceptable. Both are done here as examples. You need do only one. The quantities of vehicle must be expressed in the same unit of measurement on both sides.

(a) Convert the active ingredient either (1) from grains to milligrams or (2) from milligrams to grains.

$$\frac{60 \text{ mg}}{\text{gr i}} = \frac{x \text{ (mg)}}{\text{gr } \frac{1}{75}}$$

(1)
$$x = 60 \times \frac{1}{75}$$

$$x = \frac{4}{5} \text{ or } 0.8 \text{ mg}$$

Thus far all we have found out is that gr $\frac{1}{75}$ = 0.8 mg.

$$\frac{60 \text{ mg}}{\text{gr i}} = \frac{0.2 \text{ mg}^a}{x \text{ (gr)}}$$

$$60x = \frac{2}{10}$$

(2)
$$x = \frac{2}{10} \div 60$$

$$x = \frac{2}{10} \times \frac{1}{60}$$

$$x = \frac{2}{600} = \frac{1}{300} \text{ gr}$$

^{a} We change the decimal early, because it is easier. (We must use fractions in the apothecary system.)

Thus far we have found that 0.2 mg = gr $\frac{1}{300}$.

(b) Convert the vehicle.
   (i) Identify the quantities of measures—here cubic centimeters and drams.
   (ii) Think through the conversion equivalents that you have memorized—the established relationship between the two involved quantities—4 cc = dr 1.

(iii) Substitute dr 1 for 4 cc in the problem. We can thus express the problem in terms of mg/dr or gr/dr:

Dose available: 0.2 mg/dr (substituted for 4 cc)
Desired dose: 0.8 mg/dr _____

or

Dose available: gr $\dfrac{1}{300}$ per dr

Desired dose: gr $\dfrac{1}{75}$ per dr _____

4. We now are ready to solve the problem, either in terms of mg/dr or gr/dr.

(a)

$$\frac{0.2 \text{ mg}}{\text{dr } 1} = \frac{0.8 \text{ mg}}{(\text{dr}) \, x}$$

$$0.2x = 0.8$$

$$x = 0.8 \div 0.2$$

$$x = \text{dr } 4$$

or

$$\frac{\text{gr } \dfrac{1}{300}}{\text{dr } 1} = \frac{\text{gr } \dfrac{1}{75}}{(\text{dr}) \, x}$$

(b)

$$\frac{1}{300} x = \frac{1}{75}$$

$$x = \frac{1}{75} \div \frac{1}{300}$$

$$x = \frac{1}{75} \times 300$$

$$x = \text{dr } 4$$

Note that the different methods used yield the same answer.

▶ When you feel that you understand this material, complete Activity Sheet 5.

Activity Sheet 5

1. A liquid oral medication comes 0.25 g/dr and you wish to give gr xii. How many cc will you give?

2. There are 150 gr in a 10-cc bottle and you must administer 0.25 g. You will give _____ cc or m _____ .

3. 0.6 mg of medication are in ʒi. You must give 225 mcg. You will give ʒ _____ .

4. You must give gr xii and the medicine is available as 750 mg per ʒ ss̄. How much fluid will you give for the following:
    (a) in ʒ   (b) in cc   (c) in T   (d) in t

5. You are directed to give 1 mg of a medication and you have available gr 1/120 per cc. You will give _____ .

6. The liquids a person had for lunch consisted of 4 oz of juice, 3 t cream for jello, 100 cc of jello, and 4 T broth. What was the fluid intake in cc?

7. An oral medication is available as gr i s̄s̄ per 15 cc and you must administer 0.2 g. How much will you give in household measure?

8. A medication comes as 0.2 g per 10 cc. To give gr vii s̄s̄, how many cc will you give?

9. A drug comes as gr 1/150 per cc. You must give 0.2 mg. You will give _____ .

10. A drug comes as gr v per tablet and you must administer 600 mg. How many tablets will you give?

11. A medicine comes gr 1/4 per cc. You must administer 5 mg. You will give m _____ .

12. An oral suspension comes as gr vii s̄s̄ per ounce. How many milligrams of medication are in each 1-dr dose?

13. You must administer 250 mg of a medication. It is available as gr ii per cc. You will give _____ .

14. A medicine is available as gr xv per 8 cc. The dose you must administer is 150 mg. How many cc is this?

15. Medication is ordered as gr 3/4. It is available as 100 mg/cc. You will give _____ cc.

16. You must give gr 1/50. It is available as 0.6 mg/cc. You will give _____ cc.

17. A medicine is available as 500 mg and you must give gr vii s̄s̄. You will give _____ tablet(s).

18. A medicine is available as gr 1/2. You must give 15 mg. You will give _____ tablet(s).

19. A liquid medication comes 60 gr/oz. How many milligrams of medication are in dr 1?

20. You are ordered to give 10 mg. The drug is available as gr 1/4 per cc. You will give m _____ .

21. A medication comes gr x per cc. You must give 0.3 g. You will give _____ cc.

22. Give 100 mg. The preparation available is gr i s̄s̄ per ʒ s̄s̄. You will give ʒ _____ , ℥ _____ , _____ cc, or _____ T.

23. A drug is ordered as gr 1/12. The tablets available are 2.5 mg, 5 mg, and 0.2 mg. What size tablet and how many should be administered?

24. A medicine of 0.06 g is ordered. Available tablets are gr i s̄s̄, gr s̄s̄, and gr 1/4. What should be administered?

25. A drug comes gr s̄s̄ per cc and you must administer 7.5 mg. You will give _____ cc.

26. You must administer 12 mg. The tablets available are 4 mg, 6 mg, gr 1/5, gr 1/6, and gr 1/10. The best selection to administer is _____ tablet(s) of the _____ strength.

27. You must administer gr 1/15. The tablets available are gr 1/30, gr 1/7.5, 4 mg, 40 mg, and 15 mg. The best selection to administer is _____ tablet(s) of the _____ strength.

28. You must administer gr 1/200. The tablets available are gr 1/400, gr 1/100, 3 mg, 0.3 mg, and 3.33 mg. The best selection to administer is _____ tablet(s) of the _____ strength.

29. You must administer 0.5 mg. The tablets available are 0.125 mg, 0.25 mg, gr 1/2, gr 1/60, and gr 1/120. The best selection to administer is _____ tablet(s) of the _____ strength.

30. You have available the following tablets: 12 mg, 3 mg, gr 1/6, gr 1/10, and gr x. You must administer 6 mg. The best selection to administer is _____ tablet(s) of the _____ strength.

► Compare your answers with those at the end of this chapter. If you have answered all questions correctly, take the posttest. Otherwise, review the preceding text and correct your mistakes before taking the posttest.

Posttest

1. Conversion factors and equivalents:

(a) $\mathfrak{Z}$ = _____ cc   (b) 1 t = _____ cc

(c) m 15 to 16 = _____ cc   (d) $\mathfrak{Z}$ = _____ cc

(e) 1 t = $\mathfrak{Z}$ _____   (f) T = _____ oz

(g) T = _____ cc   (h) 1 gtt = m _____

(i) oz = $\mathfrak{Z}$ _____   (j) oz = _____ cc

(k) gr = _____ mg   (l) gr 15 = _____ g

(m) cc = _____ gtt   (n) gr 12 = _____ g

(o) 10 gr = _____ g   (p) gr 5 = _____ g

(q) 4 gr = _____ g   (r) gr 2 = _____ g

(s) gr $\dfrac{3}{4}$ = _____ mg

2. Are you able to utilize 15 and 16 m interchangeably in your calculations, depending upon which figure will make your answer come out evenly?

3. A medication comes gr $\overline{ss}$ per cc. You must administer gr 1/16. You will give m _____ .

4. You must administer 0.75 g. Your medicine is available as gr xii per 4 cc. You will give dr _____ .

5. You must administer 10 mg. You have available gr 1/3 per $\mathfrak{Z}$. You will give _____ cc.

6. You must administer gr 3/4. You have available 100 mg per 30 cc. You will give $\mathfrak{Z}$ _____ .

7. You must administer gr 45. You have 1000 mg per oz 2/3. You will give _____ cc.

8. You must give ℥ i. You have available gr x per ℥ ii. You will give _____ mg.

9. You must give 15 cc. The medicine is available as gr xv per oz. You will give _____ mg.

10. You must administer 0.25 g. You have available gr iv per t. You will give _____ cc.

11. You have available gr 1/600 per t. You must administer 0.4 mg. You will give ℥ _____ .

12. You have available gr 1/15 per 5 cc. You must administer 12 mg. You will give _____ t.

13. You have available 0.2 mg per ℥. You must administer gr 1/60. You will give _____ t.

14. You have available gr 1/5 per T. You must administer 3 mg. You will give ℥ _____ .

15. You have available gr vii $\overline{ss}$ per T. You must administer 1.5 g. You will give _____ cc.

16. You have available 0.2 mg per ℥. You must administer gr 1/50. You will give _____ T.

17. You have available 100 mg per 60 cc. You must administer gr i $\overline{ss}$. You will give _____ T.

18. You must administer gr ii. You have available 0.25 g/oz. You will give _____ cc.

19. There are 0.6 g per 60 cc. You must administer gr v. You will give ℥ _____ .

20. You have available 0.5 mg tablets. You must give gr 1/240. You will give _____ tablet(s).

21. You have available gr vii $\overline{ss}$ per tablet. You must administer 2500 mg. You will give _____ tablet(s).

22. You must administer gr 3/4. You have available 50 mg tablets. You will administer _____ tablet(s).

TPO   IPO

2   25–29,
      32

23. You must administer 7.5 mg. You have available the following tablets: 3.25 mg, 15 mg, gr 1/8, gr 1/4, and gr $\overline{ss}$. The most appropriate dose is _____ tablet(s) of the _____ strength.

2   25–29,
      32

24. You must administer gr 1/300. You have available the following tablets: gr 1/75, gr 1/150, 0.1 mg, 0.2 mg, and 0.4 mg. The most appropriate dose is _____ tablet(s) of the _____ strength.

▶   Compare your answers with those at the end of this chapter. If you have answered all questions correctly, you have successfully completed this chapter. If any of your answers were incorrect, note the objective numbers next to them, review the relevant text, complete some similar questions on the activity sheets, and correct your mistakes on this test. Then take the pretest of this chapter as a second posttest.

Answers for Chapter 15

PRETEST

1. (a) 15 to 16   (b) 4   (c) 5   (d) 30   (e) $1\frac{1}{4}$ (f) 4
   (g) 15 to 16   (h) 15   (i) 8   (j) 30   (k) 1   (l) 60
   (m) 0.75   (n) 0.6   (o) 0.3   (p) 0.12   (q) 45 to 50
   (r) 0.25   (s) 15

2. Yes   3. 2   4. 1   5. $1\frac{1}{3}$

6. 2   7. 80   8. 0.6   9. 1000
10. 5   11. 5   12. 2   13. 4

14. 2   15. 45   16. $1\frac{1}{2}$ 17. 3

18. 60   19. $\frac{1}{2}$ 20. $\frac{1}{2}$ 21. 5

22. 1   23. One, gr $\frac{1}{4}$ 24. One, 0.4 mg

ACTIVITY SHEET 1

1. 30   2. 4   3. 15 to 16   4. 30 to 32
5. ii $\overline{ss}$ 6. 4   7. 10   8. 10

9. $\overline{ss}$ 10. $\frac{2}{3}$ 11. 128   12. 105

13. 19 or xix   14. $1\frac{2}{3}$ 15. $\overline{ss}$ 16. 75

17. 10   18. i $\overline{ss}$ 19. 10   20. v
21. xxv   22. i $\overline{ss}$ 23. v   24. 1
25. i $\overline{ss}$ 26. 2 or ii   27. 0.84

372   III: USING THE APOTHECARY SYSTEM OF MEASUREMENT

ACTIVITY SHEET 2

1. 5	2. 20	3. 12	4. 10
5. 4	6. 20	7. 28	8. 4
9. 25	10. 4		

ACTIVITY SHEET 3

1. 1
2. 15 to 16
3. 4, 15
4. 1

5. 4 or iv
6. 1, 30
7. $1\frac{1}{4}$, 1
8. 10 or x

9. 9   10. 4   11. 8   12. 45
13. 1   14. 5   15. 75   16. 16
17. 150   18. 240   19. 5   20. 2 t

21. 3   22. 1   23. 110   24. $83\frac{1}{3}$ mg

25. 15 to 16 gtt   26. 1 t   27. $1\frac{1}{2}$ T

28. 2 t   29. $\frac{1}{2}$

ACTIVITY SHEET 4

1. (a) If the quantity you are converting is gr 1 (60 mg) or less, use the equivalent 60 mg = gr 1.
   (b) If the quantity you are converting is more than 1 gr (60 mg), use the equivalent gr 15 = 1 g (1000 mg).
2. gr xii = 750 mg (0.75 g)
   gr x = 600 mg (0.6 g)
   gr 5 = 300 mg (0.3 g)
   gr 4 = 250 mg (0.25 g)
   gr 2 = 120 mg (0.12 g)
   gr $\frac{3}{4}$ = 50 or 45 mg

3. 0.75, 12   4. 15   5. $\frac{3}{10}$ (0.3)   6. $\frac{2}{5}$ (0.4)
7. 1   8. 250   9. 0.1, i $\overline{ss}$ 10. 30
11. 2   12. 0.3, 300   13. 0.5, 500   14. 1; 1000
15. $\frac{2}{3}$ 16. $\frac{1}{8}$ 17. $\frac{1}{120}$ 18. $\frac{3}{4}$
19. 45 or 50   20. $\frac{1}{6}$

ACTIVITY SHEET 5

1. 12   2. $\frac{1}{4}$, 4   3. 3

4. 4, 15, 1, 3   5. 2 cc   6. 295
7. 1 oz or 2 T   8. 25   9. 0.5 cc
10. 2   11. 5   12. 62.5   13. 2 cc
14. 1.2   15. 0.5   16. 2   17. 1
18. $\frac{1}{2}$ 19. 500   20. 10   21. 0.5

22. $\overline{ss}$, 4, 15, 1 T   23. One of the 5 mg tablets
24. Two of the gr $\overline{ss}$ tablets

25. $\frac{1}{4}$ (0.25)   26. One of the gr $\frac{1}{5}$ tablets

27. One of the 4 mg   28. One of the 0.3 mg

29. One of the gr $\frac{1}{120}$ 30. One of the gr $\frac{1}{10}$

POSTTEST

1. (a) 4   (b) 5   (c) 1   (d) 30   (e) $1\frac{1}{4}$ (f) $\frac{1}{2}$ (g) 15

   (h) 1   (i) 8   (j) 30   (k) 60   (l) 1   (m) 15 to 16
   (n) 0.75   (o) 0.6   (p) 0.3   (q) 0.25   (r) 0.12 (s) 45 or 50
2. Yes   3. 2   4. 1   5. 2
6. $\frac{1}{2}$ 7. 60   8. 300   9. 500
10. 5   11. 5   12. 3   13. 4
14. 1   15. 45   16. $1\frac{1}{2}$ 17. 4
18. 15   19. 1   20. $\frac{1}{2}$ (0.5)   21. 5
22. 1   23. One gr $\frac{1}{8}$ tablet
24. One 0.2 mg tablet